# THE NEW
# HOSPITAL–
# PHYSICIAN
# ENTERPRISE

## MEETING THE CHALLENGES
## OF VALUE-BASED CARE

# THE NEW
# HOSPITAL–
# PHYSICIAN
# ENTERPRISE

## MEETING THE CHALLENGES
## OF VALUE-BASED CARE

David A. Wofford and Stephen F. Messinger, Editors

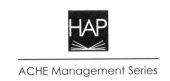

ACHE Management Series

Your board, staff, or clients may also benefit from this book's insight. For more information on quantity discounts, contact the Health Administration Press Marketing Manager at (312) 424-9470.

This publication is intended to provide accurate and authoritative information in regard to the subject matter covered. It is sold, or otherwise provided, with the understanding that the publisher is not engaged in rendering professional services. If professional advice or other expert assistance is required, the services of a competent professional should be sought.

The statements and opinions contained in this book are strictly those of the authors and do not represent the official positions of the American College of Healthcare Executives or the Foundation of the American College of Healthcare Executives.

17   16   15   14          5   4   3   2

Library of Congress Cataloging-in-Publication Data

The new hospital–physician enterprise : meeting the challenges of value-based care / David A. Wofford and Stephen F. Messinger, editors.
    pages cm
 Includes index.
 ISBN 978-1-56793-598-1 (alk. paper)
 1.  Hospital-physician relations. 2.  Hospital-physician joint ventures. 3.  Medical care—Cost effectiveness. I. Wofford, David A., editor of compilation. II. Messinger, Stephen F., editor of compilation
 RA971.9.N49 2013
 362.11—dc23
                     2013011313

The paper used in this publication meets the minimum requirements of American National Standard for Information Sciences—Permanence of Paper for Printed Library Materials, ANSI Z39.48-1984. ∞ ™

Acquisitions editor: Janet Davis; Project manager: Andrew Baumann; Cover designer: Marisa Jackson; Layout: Cepheus Edmondson

Found an error or a typo? We want to know! Please e-mail it to hapbooks@ache.org, and put "Book Error" in the subject line.

For photocopying and copyright information, please contact Copyright Clearance Center at www.copyright.com or at (978) 750-8400.

Health Administration Press
A division of the Foundation of the American
   College of Healthcare Executives
One North Franklin Street, Suite 1700
Chicago, IL 60606-3529
(312) 424-2800

# Contents

## Part I: Integrated Models

## Part II: Alternative Alignment Models

## Part III: Special Considerations

# Preface

## THE CHALLENGE

The US healthcare industry differs from any other industry in the world in some fundamental and alarming ways. It is huge and is fast approaching $3 trillion in expenditures annually (CMS 2013). It is fragmented, with hundreds of thousands of providers and facilities most often operating as independent businesses. It lacks performance standards, with little agreement regarding what constitutes high-quality care and how to improve outcomes. The consumers and providers who decide what services are provided are largely insulated from the cost of those services, which is borne by government and employers.

The results of these structural issues—lack of coordination, inability to define quality or efficacy of care, and misalignment of economic incentives—are by now recognized not only by those in the industry but by the general public as well. Costs have risen to unsustainable levels, with little evidence that people in the United States are any better off than residents of countries that spend a substantially smaller percentage of their GDP on healthcare. It is no surprise that we are witnessing an unprecedented movement, driven largely by these escalating costs, toward reforming both the organization and the financing of healthcare.

The challenge, of course, is that many provider organizations are ill equipped to adapt to the level of change that is required for this reform. As much as we like to talk about constant change being a way of life, the reality is that most healthcare provider organizations have enjoyed stability and a relatively benign competitive marketplace. By contrast, we need only consider the radical transformations that the banking, media, and consumer retail industries underwent following the advent of the Internet. Because of the stability that has existed in healthcare, nimbleness and innovation have not been necessities and therefore have not generally been developed as core capabilities.

As healthcare reimbursement shifts from volume- to value-based models, hospitals and physicians are under increasing pressure to work together. Clearly, providers will increasingly be rewarded for efficiency and outcomes of care (i.e., value), and hospitals need to place high priority on alignment with physicians to accommodate the coming changes in payment mechanisms. The success of healthcare organizations will depend on their ability to bring hospitals, physicians, and other providers together to improve the quality of care while reducing total costs. Unfortunately, many are discovering that hospital–physician alignment is difficult to achieve, and increasingly so in the post-reform world. With notable exceptions, hospitals have historically tended to shy away from forming close alignment with physicians unless lucrative inpatient referrals were at stake. In the future, however, financial incentives will be radically transformed, and hospitals need to rethink how they approach their physician relationships.

For many organizations, hospital–physician alignment feels like uncharted territory. The purpose of this book is to provide in-depth information about creating and sustaining an economically integrated physician component within a larger health system.

## PREREQUISITES FOR SUCCESS

Given the significant challenges ahead, certain characteristics are important for success as an integrated provider of healthcare services. From our work with organizations at varying degrees of readiness, the following themes are emerging:

- **Ability to define a vision for the future:** Many readers will recall how, while preparing for his 1992 campaign, President George H. W. Bush famously dismissed "the vision thing" and then went on to lose what should have been a relatively easy reelection against the less established but more eloquent challenger, Bill Clinton. The parallel between presidential politics and healthcare is not often drawn but is fitting in this case. Healthcare leaders have been primarily focused on operational issues, often to the detriment of strategic concerns. However, in a time when the environment truly is changing, healthcare leaders must increasingly be aware of regional and national developments, interpret them appropriately, identify the correct organizational response, and then communicate that response clearly and convincingly to their constituents.

- **Willingness to let go of the status quo:** Defining a vision for the future is one thing; seeing it through is another. One of the most common stumbling blocks is that the culture of independent hospitals and physicians stubbornly resists change. Too often, healthcare leaders say they want to set a new course and achieve alignment between hospitals and physicians, when the reality is that they want things to stay fundamentally the same. Organizations that are successful at physician alignment have leaders who recognize that they must share control with physicians, develop innovative contracting approaches, transform their clinical and business processes, and publish information on quality and outcomes.

- **Capital to invest in the physician enterprise:** With very few exceptions, hospitals and health systems that want to align with physicians in a meaningful way will end up acquiring at least some of those physicians' practices as well as recruiting new physicians into the enterprise. Most often, physicians will be employed, but the enterprise may also include "employment-like" models involving professional services agreements, such as are common in states with more stringent corporate-practice-of-medicine statutes. Capital requirements go far beyond the initial outlay for the acquisition itself and include money for starting up new practices, supporting ongoing operational deficits, and building the infrastructure needed to coordinate care and demonstrate value.
- **Physician practice management expertise:** As we discuss in this book, the integrated enterprise must be well versed in managing physician practices, because the consequences of poor management can be ruinous to an organization that is already operating on thin margins and facing large capital requirements. This type of expertise is not easily learned on the job; the integrated enterprise requires professional management by individuals who understand physician performance metrics, compensation, revenue cycle, and so forth.

Because not every hospital or health system has all of the above capabilities, success at achieving meaningful alignment with physicians will be beyond the reach of some organizations as they are currently structured. For those organizations, we see two paths, both of which are occurring with increasing frequency.[1] The first is to merge with another organization or organizations and pool the capabilities outlined above (or develop them together). Rather than being the primary integrator, the organizations that take this first path will be partners or subsidiaries of an existing hospital-based integrator.

The second path is for the hospital to provide inpatient services under contract to another entity or entities. This entity could be a hospital-based system, a medical group, or a health insurance company. We see this arrangement—the hospital as a vendor of services—in several markets already. For example, Group Health Cooperative in Washington State has made the strategic decision to exit the hospital business altogether and instead contract with several hospitals in its service area for inpatient services. Similarly, several independent practice associations in Southern California are accepting inpatient insurance risk and contracting for these services through local hospitals. In both cases, these organizations provide inpatient services through contracts with area hospitals without taking on the financial commitment of owning and operating hospitals.

Most organizations would rather be the dominant party in integration efforts, but many (in fact, most) hospitals will either be a part of someone else's system or serve as a vendor of hospital services to one or more unaffiliated systems. Although a hospital may have difficulty accepting that these are its best available options, the hospital must pursue strategies that reflect this reality.

## HOW IT WILL PLAY OUT

To be sure, many unknowns await healthcare providers in the foreseeable future. To develop an effective response—to the extent this is possible—healthcare leaders must have reasonable expectations regarding how events will unfold. We anticipate the following trends:

- **Industry consolidation will continue.** The trend toward consolidation within the healthcare industry will continue well into the foreseeable future and will include both horizontal (e.g., hospital–hospital) and vertical (e.g., hospital–physician, payer–hospital, payer–physician) consolidation. A wide range of factors will drive this consolidation, including the need to succeed under value-based reimbursement; physicians' desire to practice within large, established organizations rather than in small, private practices; and the inevitable failure of some organizations to succeed as integrated entities. Although consolidation is widely recognized as a necessary precondition for healthcare reform to succeed, how fully it will be accepted by the agencies charged with antitrust regulatory enforcement remains to be seen. Our expectation is that developing appropriate regulations will be a slow and frustrating process, regardless of the political climate.
- **New healthcare organizations will emerge.** Hospitals have been the dominant focus of integration in the past, primarily because they have had both the capital and the management needed to acquire medical practices and negotiate with payers. Hospitals have not, however, been nimble innovators. Driven by payment reform, the need for scale, and competitive pressures, more entrepreneurial models will appear with frequency. These models will range from narrow networks created by health insurers to accountable care organizations (ACOs) developed by large physician groups to partnerships between providers, insurers, and financiers. Hospitals and health systems will have to find ways to be at the table when these arrangements are being developed.
- **Private practice will shrink.** More than half of all physicians in the United States now belong to hospital-owned practices. We are seeing no slowdown in the pace of this transition, and we believe that the era of the independent private practice as we know it is drawing to a close. The few physicians who

remain in private practice will be either in small subspecialties or unsuited, for a variety of reasons, for work in a large, bureaucratic organization. Most physicians will seek employment in integrated systems and large medical groups for reasons other than the fact that it is a better model; an increasing number of physicians simply do not want to be in private practice, where they have to be small business owners as well as clinicians, and many hospitals will need to employ physicians to meet the community's needs or to prevent them from working for the competition.

- **Specialty physician compensation will change.** Changes in reimbursement will have a major impact on the economics of various specialty practices, with a resulting redistribution of physician compensation. We expect that ancillary margins will continue to decline, advantageous 340B pricing for chemotherapy drugs may be revisited, and incentives for managing the continuum of care will be increased. As a result, primary care physicians and hospitalists will be in even greater demand, and their compensation will increase accordingly. Specialists, particularly those whose incomes have historically been driven by ancillaries such as cardiology, oncology, and some surgical specialties, will see relatively smaller compensation increases. Further, broader use of evidence-based medicine protocols may lessen the volume of tests and procedures, limiting the revenue generated by specialists. Compensation will change only incrementally over time, because many employed physicians' compensation arrangements are based on published benchmarks and tend to reinforce those benchmarks. Moving forward, physician compensation methodologies should reflect the new paradigm of value-based reimbursement rather than the production-based systems that are being replaced.

## ABOUT THIS BOOK

This book is organized into three parts. Part I addresses issues that are common to integrated models. *Integrated* refers to employment or employment-like[2] models in which the hospital or health system owns the clinic assets, employs the staff, and manages the physician practice. Part I begins with a discussion of the correct mind-set and expectations prior to acquiring physician practices and then moves on to explain managing an acquisition, building effective physician leadership, compensating physicians, and managing operations and revenue cycle. In Part II, we address several alignment models in which physicians continue to maintain practices independent of the hospital or health system. In particular, these models include clinical joint ventures, clinical comanagement arrangements, ACOs, and the use of information technology. Finally, in Part III, we address two topics that are applicable to both integrated and more loosely affiliated models: fair market value and payer contracting strategies.

Creating this book has been a major undertaking, but for us it has been a labor of love because it reflects many years spent addressing interesting and important issues in collaboration with organizations that we respect and admire. We hope the reader will find it relevant and informative.

David A. Wofford
Stephen F. Messinger

## NOTES

1. A potential third path is to serve as a major referral center for highly special-ized services, such as organ transplant, with more traditional hospital–physi-cian relationships and payer contracts. However, this option is not realistic for the vast majority of hospitals and health systems.
2. For example, in states where corporate-practice-of-medicine laws exist, profes-sional services agreements are commonly structured with nonemployed physi-cians, who provide physician services in outpatient facilities that are owned and operated by the hospital or health system.

## REFERENCE

Centers for Medicare & Medicaid Services (CMS). 2013. "National Health Expenditures Projections 2011–2012." Accessed February 12. www.cms .gov/Research-Statistics-Data-and-Systems/Statistics-Trends-and-Reports/ NationalHealthExpendData/Downloads/Proj2011PDF.pdf.

# Acknowledgments

Writing this book has been a major undertaking and has involved many people who are connected to ECG Management Consultants, Inc., in addition to the named authors. Their contributions were invaluable, and without their assistance, getting this book to print would have proved significantly more challenging. We would like to take this opportunity to acknowledge their efforts.

The following consultants and content experts from ECG assisted in developing the book:

- Gita B. Budd and Brian J. Orgen—physician strategy of health systems
- Maria C. Hayduk and Jamaal A. Campbell—physician compensation plan development
- Jason R. Peterson, Todd W. Godfrey, Erin R. Gosney, and Miranda Mooneyham—medical practice operational performance
- Amanda P. Tosto, RN—integrated systems and accountable care organizations
- Claudie D. Bolduc—alternative models to physician employment, including joint ventures and clinical comanagement arrangements
- Rebecca L. Levy—fair market value considerations
- Purvi B. Bhatt, Charles A. Brown, and Katie C. Fellin—accountable care organizations and payment reform implications
- Laura D. Jantos—use of IT as an integration strategy
- Robert G. Rowland—tireless coaching, cajoling, and assisting the authors in developing and polishing their chapter content

In addition, Chris A. Clarke, RN, CMPE, LSSBB, a friend of the firm, contributed material and assisted with the writing by providing a "view from the trenches," which gave invaluable insight regarding the mind-set of physicians and hospital leadership working together post-integration.

Finally, the following stars of ECG's administrative team did a fabulous job of keeping us on track:

- Cassandra J. Greenwald, editor, who maintained ECG's editorial standards for all content
- Sandra Gelb, manager of our document production center, who created the file repository and maintained version control
- Kathryn A. Sweyer, marketing manager, who managed the overall execution of this project

# Part I

# INTEGRATED MODELS

# CHAPTER 1

# Begin with the End in Mind

*Francine D. Merenghi and David A. Wofford*

THE HEALTHCARE INDUSTRY has recently seen a dramatic increase in activity related to hospital–physician alignment, with the most notable changes occurring in the acquisition of physician practices. Typically, practice acquisition means physician employment, although employment-like models also exist in which the medical group remains a separate legal entity, such as medical foundations (particularly in states that have corporate-practice-of-medicine prohibitions). In the interest of simplicity, this chapter treats both models as employment arrangements.

Regardless of the type of arrangement, hospitals often feel pressure to acquire practices quickly, either because they face direct competition from other hospitals in acquiring those practices or because the physicians are anxious, for a host of reasons, to sell their practices. Unfortunately, in the rush to get the deal done, longer-term planning around the hospital–physician relationship tends to take a backseat to the urgent demands of completing the transaction. Thinking in terms of the transactional versus relational elements of the arrangement is therefore useful (Exhibit 1.1).

Ideally, the discussions between the hospital and the physicians would strike an appropriate balance between transactional considerations and the relational elements that focus on how physicians and hospital leadership will work together postintegration. The challenge is to take the time to define and establish these relational elements before the deal is done, rather than deferring these difficult decisions until later. If issues are left open or subject to interpretation by either party, they are likely to emerge during times of stress—for example, when the organization is struggling with operational changes or financial losses. By then, however, both the physicians and the hospital will be frustrated and will invariably find it much more difficult to introduce, discuss, and resolve problems in their relationship. When

**Exhibit 1.1  Transactional Versus Relational Considerations of Practice Integration**

| Transactional Considerations | Relational Considerations |
| --- | --- |
| Financial analysis | Vision |
| Asset valuations | Leadership and management |
| Due diligence | Decision making |
| Compensation and benefits | Culture |
| Legal document preparation | Communication |
| Lease and contract assignments | Medical staff relationships |
| Day 1 operational provisions | Joint strategic planning |

the acquisition occurs prior to the planning, the integrated entity can find itself in a difficult position (Exhibit 1.2).

Obviously, this path is a painful one to follow. Taking a more effective approach provides opportunity for a long-term, stable relationship between the hospital and employed physicians. The key is to commit to a comprehensive planning process prior to engaging in acquisition or employment negotiations. This planning process will build the foundation for a highly successful and healthy long-term relationship with physician partners. The ideal path includes three phases—planning and strategy, business development, and execution (Exhibit 1.3). The remainder of this chapter focuses on the first two phases of this development path. The third phase, execution, is addressed in Chapter 5.

**Exhibit 1.2  Typical Development Path (Practices Acquired Prior to Planning)**

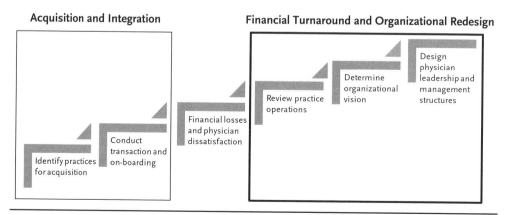

Acquisition and Integration

Financial Turnaround and Organizational Redesign

Identify practices for acquisition

Conduct transaction and on-boarding

Financial losses and physician dissatisfaction

Review practice operations

Determine organizational vision

Design physician leadership and management structures

**Exhibit 1.3 Desired Development Path (Practices Acquired After Planning)**

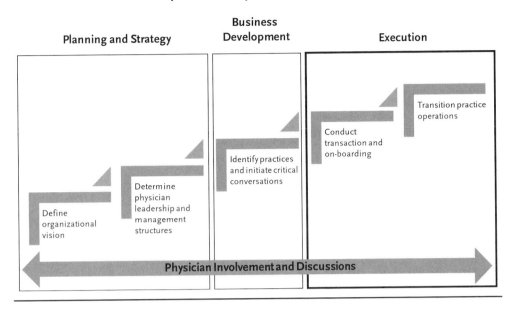

Defining the physician alignment approach and establishing key elements of the health system employment strategy—such as physician leadership, compensation philosophy, and management infrastructure—are critical first steps a hospital needs to take before entering into more detailed employment discussions with physicians.

Although the first two phases of the planning process are internal to the health system, involving medical staff leadership in these discussions is crucial. Doing so engages key physician leaders in strategic thinking and can also help mitigate potential negative reactions from independent medical staff members later. During these first two phases, using a third-party facilitator to keep the conversations on track and to achieve desired objectives can sometimes be beneficial.

## PHASE I: PLAN FOR SUCCESS

### Start with a Vision

If a hospital wants to employ physicians on anything more than a strictly ad hoc, opportunistic basis, the hospital must begin with a clear understanding of what the physician enterprise is intended to accomplish and how it fits into the larger organization. For most hospitals, this means developing a strategy that redefines the organization as an integrated health system rather than a hospital-centric entity that just so happens to employ physicians. In the absence of such a strategy, the tendency is usually to treat the physician practices as little more than a hospital department or ancillary business—which may result in some degree of tactical success, such as stabilizing a portion of the medical staff or providing a needed service that the community could not support in private practice, but not much more. Therefore, hospitals must dedicate sufficient time up front to set the tone of the relationship, form the foundation of the health system's employment strategy, and establish the guiding principles for a successful, long-term relationship. Typically, the physician strategy is informed by the larger strategic goals of the healthcare system; without a solid understanding of what the system is trying to accomplish, the physician strategy cannot be tailored to support the vision of the larger entity. In developing its strategy, the hospital should explicitly address several topics (see Exhibit 1.4 for examples).

## Plan for a Common Culture

Hospitals or health systems sometimes assume that employed physicians will conform to their culture and behavioral expectations. However, this assumption is dangerous, for a variety of reasons. Physicians are trained to think and act independently and are usually not inclined to modify the way they do things simply because their employment arrangement has changed. Whereas the first loyalty of administrators is usually to the organization, physicians may have many loyalties, including to their patients, to their fellow physicians, and perhaps only then to the organization. Additionally, physicians are fully aware that the hospital's business model is completely dependent on the patient–physician relationship, and they will be protective of this relationship. Without up-front relationship building and discussion of expectations, employment of physicians will not result in a more integrated or unified relationship. Many health system managers have difficulty understanding that employed physicians don't wear the home-team colors just because they are employed.

To achieve a more stable and successful partnership, the physician enterprise should be regarded as an integral part of the organization, on an equal footing with the hospital. Success is difficult, if not impossible, to achieve if the hospital treats physicians as rank-and-file employees and tries to impose existing policies, procedures, and culture on them. Instead, a more effective approach allows a blended culture to emerge that respects the physician perspective and involves physicians in decision making at all levels of the organization. This approach requires hospital senior management to accept that it must change and share decision-making power, and that this change can actually be beneficial.

**Exhibit 1.4  Key Questions When Planning the Physician Enterprise**

| Key Question | Potential Answers |
|---|---|
| What do we want to achieve? | ◆ Performance under risk-based contracts<br>◆ Geographic expansion<br>◆ Meeting of community need for specialty-specific services<br>◆ Succession for aging medical staff<br>◆ Strengthening of market position<br>◆ Stabilization of the medical community |
| How extensively will we employ physicians? | ◆ On an opportunistic basis only<br>◆ As a key feature of our strategy<br>◆ As the definition of who we are |
| How will we define success? | ◆ Physician recruitment and retention<br>◆ Expansion of services and locations<br>◆ Improvement in clinical quality measures<br>◆ Financial performance relative to budget |
| How will the physician enterprise be organized and governed? | ◆ Physician-led and professionally managed<br>◆ Physician division or enterprise<br>◆ Provider-based designation |

## Include Physicians in Management

Hospitals that employ physicians should actively seek ways to tap into physicians' knowledge and expertise by involving them in the management of the organization. For a hospital to achieve the goals identified during the early planning and strategy sessions, the missing link can be the involvement of physician partners who are committed to the organization, understand patient care, and have shared incentives. Physicians who seek employment generally want to shape their future, and many of them are anxious to take on leadership roles and facilitate better coordination of patient care in the community. Shared decision making does not often come naturally to hospital executives, who tend to be risk averse and believe their job is to maintain control over all aspects of the organization's strategic direction and operations. In some cases, this risk aversion may be fueled by a need to avoid upsetting the independent members of the medical staff, who may feel threatened by the prospect of employed physicians holding leadership positions within the physician enterprise or health system.

These concerns are valid, but to realize the full benefits of integration, physicians and hospital executives must acknowledge that the integrated organization has a much broader scope of activity, encompassing inpatient and outpatient care, for a larger and more varied population than either party has served in the past. Addressing this larger scope is difficult even for the most advanced systems. To be successful, hospitals and physicians need to recognize that each party brings critical and unique skills to the table and that these skills should be respected and nurtured. Shared decision making leverages the strength of both clinical and administrative leadership and will promote physician satisfaction and unity. It can also facilitate accountability and engagement of physician leaders. Most important, physician leadership is needed to influence physician behavior that will lead to quality improvement—a primary goal of integration. Additional information on specific leadership and management structures involving physicians is provided in Chapter 3.

## Understand the Economic and Operational Realities

When defining its vision, the hospital must understand how an acquired physician network will affect the integrated organization. The hospital should be prepared to accept many operational realities that it may not have anticipated. The following are some examples:

* **Erosion of payer mix:** Following the acquisition, the employed physicians' payer mix will likely shift away from commercially insured patients and toward Medicare, Medicaid, and self-pay. Because most employed physician compensation plans are based on work relative value units (RVUs) and thus are payer neutral, physicians are insulated from the economics of their payer mix and therefore may become more willing to accept these patients than when they were in private practice—especially within health systems that require their employed physicians to treat all patients regardless of payer. Furthermore, independent community physicians frequently begin referring these patients to their health system–employed colleagues.
* **Decline in physician productivity:** A decrease in physician productivity is not uncommon when physicians become employed. In many cases, the decrease is a direct result of compensation arrangements that include a large salary component or guaranteed income amount. Another reason is that when physicians accept employment by the hospital, they typically are able to negotiate higher compensation levels for themselves. Even if the compensation is structured with appropriate incentives, many physicians may determine that under the new, more generous compensation arrangements, they can earn

acceptable levels of income without having to produce as much. An additional factor that can lower physician productivity is the previously mentioned change in payer mix. Physicians, in particular those in primary care, often find that the increase in Medicare, Medicaid, and uninsured patients requires more physician–patient time because this population is more complex, in terms of both acuity and social factors that affect their health. Finally, lower physician productivity can result from new work-flow processes introduced to the practice staff by the health system. These new processes could be driven by electronic health record (EHR) adoption, accreditation requirements, and hospital policies and procedures. If staff are less efficient as they adjust to a new work flow, this slowdown can affect physician productivity. Obviously, ensuring that the new processes are really required and add value to the patient visit should be an important consideration.

- **Greater infrastructure costs:** Infrastructure requirements are typically greater for hospital-owned practices than for private practices. Most acquired practices will need to be transitioned to the hospital's practice management and EHR systems, which is costly not only as a hard-dollar investment but also in terms of lost physician productivity during the transition period. Most private practices have little or no compliance infrastructure, yet in a hospital-owned environment, this infrastructure is essential and requires specialized skills. Similarly, an effective revenue cycle operation calls for a level of management and a decision support and reporting infrastructure that are seldom encountered in private practice and will therefore have to be developed. Health system–driven infrastructure requirements—for example, meeting accreditation standards or transitioning to and administering provider-based billing—are a source of added costs. More significant are new cost allocations for system-wide shared services, such as information systems, human resources, finance, facilities, legal, and risk and compliance. These allocations can add a layer of cost that does not exist in private practice.

- **Higher staff salaries and benefit costs:** Salaries and benefit costs typically increase when practices are transitioned to hospital ownership. Because hospitals' benefit plans are almost always more robust than those provided by private practice physicians, transitioning physicians and staff to the hospital's benefit plan usually involves substantial incremental costs. A less obvious impact is that most hospitals allocate benefit costs as a standard percentage of direct compensation, and the high income of physicians results in significant increases in allocated (versus actual) benefit costs. Although hospitals tend to have higher pay scales for staff, higher staff salaries are not always a fact of life. For instance, nurses typically earn less in the clinic setting than in the hospital setting. In some cases, the practice nursing staff is even accreted to the hospital's bargaining unit, an arrangement that has a significant impact on wages.

Developing realistic financial projections that factor in the post-acquisition realities is the best way to manage the expectations of hospital leadership and physicians. At the same time, the health system leadership absolutely must view these economic and operational realities in the broader context of the strategic importance of the alignment.

## Get the Right Talent

Health system leadership may be tempted to identify a bright, promising hospital administrator to manage the physician enterprise in addition to her other hospital responsibilities. A word of caution: Managing a physician enterprise requires a different skill set and perspective than does managing a hospital or even a hospital outpatient department. Physicians need to believe that their administrators speak their language and understand their world. The person leading the physician enterprise should be an experienced practice administrator and well versed in all of the practice's operational and staff functions. Certain areas of vulnerability pose challenges for physician practices, and a seasoned administrator will recognize warning signs early on. Areas of vulnerability include the following:

◆ **Physician productivity and compensation:** An environment must be created in which productivity can be optimized while compensation levels are sustained and compliance risk is avoided. See Chapter 4 for further information on this topic.

◆ **Revenue cycle:** Stringent compliance rules regarding physician billing and coding require expert oversight. The higher-volume, lower-dollar physician office–based claims receive less attention and follow-up when they are managed by a hospital's accounts receivable team, which leads to lower collections. See Chapter 6 for further information on this topic.

◆ **Ongoing clinic operations:** Hospital operations leaders lack an understanding of medical practice operations, benchmarks, and performance metrics and often try to apply hospital metrics to the physician practice. This misapplication can leave important practice metrics unmonitored and negative trends unrecognized until the problem has become significant. See Chapter 5 for further information on this topic.

- **Office-based staffing:** Staffing requirements and scope of practice are different in an office than in an acute care setting. When this distinction is not understood at a management level, it can affect staffing levels and physician productivity.

A professional practice manager will understand which performance and productivity metrics are relevant to physician practice operations and will know how to work with physicians to achieve appropriate performance levels. Recruiting an individual who has worked in a mature, integrated health system and who can bring experience and knowledge to the position will help avoid the pitfalls along the journey.

## PHASE II: BUSINESS DEVELOPMENT

### Develop a Structured Approach for Hiring

Having established the overarching strategy for physician employment and the management and organizational structure under which the physicians will operate, hospital leadership needs to develop effective policies, procedures, and infrastructure to execute on practice acquisitions. In the absence of such policies and procedures, acquisitions tend to be a series of one-off transactions, each unique and with inconsistent terms. One common misstep is to use individualized (non-standard) employment contracts, which introduce a variety of employment terms and compensation arrangements. Not only are individualized contracts extremely challenging to administer, but the lack of consistency is soon discovered by the physicians, who can quickly become dissatisfied because most will assume they are being shortchanged while others are getting a better deal. This inconsistency and ensuing dissatisfaction are particularly detrimental to efforts to build a cohesive group of employed physicians.

In many cases, the hospital ends up with practices it should never have acquired in the first place, because the implications weren't properly thought through or because the lack of a standard approach and evaluation criteria makes it harder to walk away when there is not a fit between the practice and the larger organization. This situation can be mitigated by establishing criteria for determining whether there is a fit. These criteria need to be established in advance, within the context of a well-constructed plan and without a particular acquisition in mind, so that they will be untainted by the "tyranny of the urgent." Of course, maintaining the organizational discipline to abide by these criteria is also essential. The criteria should be documented in writing and referred to faithfully before, during, and after every practice acquisition so that they are never forgotten or ignored. To that end, creating a formal assessment tool to evaluate the rationale for each acquisition is helpful. Exhibit 1.5 provides examples of criteria for evaluating whether a physician or practice would make a good partner.

## Develop a Compensation Philosophy

A properly structured compensation methodology is essential to building a well-functioning physician enterprise. This methodology begins by establishing the organization's philosophy regarding physician compensation during the planning and strategy phase and ends with designing a compensation plan (discussed in Chapter 4). A compensation philosophy is a statement of principles that will serve to communicate how the health system intends to address physician compensation; this philosophy will ultimately guide the development of a compensation plan. A reasonable compensation philosophy might include the following guiding principles:

◆ Median compensation for median work effort
◆ Emphasis on and incentives for individual productivity
◆ Payer neutrality
◆ Incentives based on outcomes, quality performance, behavior, and group citizenship
◆ Income protection for specialties that are needed to sustain a minimum number of specialists in the community
◆ A common compensation structure across all specialties wherever possible
◆ Compensation that is easily understandable and reasonable to administer

These principles do not address the details of how compensation will be calculated, but they do provide physicians with a reasonable understanding of what to expect if they become employed by the health system. Establishing a compensation philosophy in advance will help in the development of the right compensation plan.

In addition to structuring appropriate incentives, health systems should strive to maintain as much consistency as possible within the compensation methodology. Obviously, there is no one-size-fits-all formula, and some variation in methodology for certain specialties is needed to ensure that market-based compensation is provided across the board. Typically, this variation is accomplished by tying compensation to appropriate benchmarks, such as specialty-specific compensation

**Exhibit 1.5  Physician or Practice Evaluation Criteria**

| Criterion | Questions to Ask |
|---|---|
| Quality | ◆ What do the medical staff say about the physician's skills?<br>◆ Is the physician a clinical leader? Is she well respected among peers?<br>◆ What is the group's malpractice history?<br>◆ How busy is the practice? What are the practice's sources of referrals, and how long has the practice had those sources?<br>◆ What does a chart review reveal about clinical quality? |
| Success in private practice | ◆ Has there been unusually high staff turnover?<br>◆ How successful has the practice been in hiring and retaining top physician talent?<br>◆ What payer contract terms has the practice been able to negotiate?<br>◆ What does the physician compensation history reveal? How competitive are compensation levels?<br>◆ How does the practice compare to national benchmarks for best practices? |
| Citizenship | ◆ How actively do group members participate in medical staff or hospital leadership activities? Do they show evidence of thinking beyond themselves?<br>◆ What is the potential for practice members to create a positive influence on their fellow physicians?<br>◆ How well do the physicians get along with one another and with community physicians?<br>◆ How easy or difficult are the physicians to deal with? |
| Strategic fit | ◆ What is the hospital's strategic need for this specialty?<br>◆ Does the business case justify the acquisition?<br>◆ What other alignment models might satisfy both parties' needs?<br>◆ How will the independent physicians react to this acquisition? |
| Retirement horizon | ◆ What are the physicians' retirement plans? Will they be with the organization long enough to make the acquisition worthwhile?<br>◆ What is the succession plan for the senior partners?<br>◆ How critical is the retiring physicians' involvement in transitioning their patients to new physicians? |

per work RVU. Tying compensation to benchmarks does not work in all cases, however, particularly with hospital-based specialties such as anesthesiology or critical care, which do not generate their own patient volumes and are based largely on the hospital's coverage needs.

That said, preventing the unnecessary proliferation of compensation methodologies that lack a consistent, overarching design is critical. Keeping methodologies to a minimum can be difficult and requires considerable managerial discipline, because there will always be reasons, some of them valid, why a given group of physicians should have its own compensation plan. Allowing compensation methodologies to proliferate not only creates a difficult administrative burden; it also breeds disunity and distrust among the physicians.

## Manage Physician Expectations from the Outset

The manner in which physician practices are acquired and integrated will set the tone of the relationship for a long time to come. Unfortunately, this transition is often not a smooth one from the physicians' perspective. Just as things change for the hospital, physicians' lives will change dramatically as a result of integration.

Ultimately, making physicians understand things will change is the hospital's responsibility. While the physicians have a level of responsibility to conduct their own due diligence and ask the right questions, many physicians have little experience in selling their practices and need to be guided through the process. Because physicians' business acumen and sophistication vary tremendously, some may not think to ask about any number of topics. Therefore, helping physicians make an informed decision about integration so they are realistic about the extent of change—and not overpromising—will pay dividends by creating a sound foundation for the future relationship. The way to manage physicians' expectations is by being open and frank with them about these matters in the early stages of the discussions. Without effective, frequent communication, physicians can inadvertently be given false expectations about what it means to be an employed physician. They may wrongly assume that little will change under the new arrangement and that they will retain roughly the same level of autonomy they enjoyed in private practice. This expectation can play out through a myriad of unpleasant surprises relating to staffing decisions, productivity or work schedule expectations, capital allocation, compliance, and so forth.

Both sides should go out of their way to fully disclose their future vision as well as their commitments to, and expectations of, the other party. Formalizing this process by drafting a compact between the hospital and physicians to document the agreement would even be reasonable. Drafting a compact takes time and may be difficult when the pressure is on to get the deal done, but addressing issues sooner rather than later will make life much easier for both parties and will set the tone for how issues should be resolved after integration takes place. In some cases, scheduling a facilitated retreat may ensure that sufficient time and attention are dedicated to developing a common understanding of how the parties will function as an integrated entity. Exhibit 1.6 outlines some key areas that should be discussed and decided early on in the process. Each of these issues needs to be discussed in the context of an integrated health system and not solely from a hospital-centric or physician-centric point of view.

For this communication to be effective, close coordination between the individuals charged with negotiating the transaction and those who will ultimately manage day-to-day practice operations is important. If these functions exist in

**Exhibit 1.6 Key Integration Topics of Discussion**

| Area | Topic |
|------|-------|
| Organization | ◆ Organizational and management structure of the physician enterprise<br>◆ Degree of decision-making authority delegated to the physician enterprise<br>◆ Roles of the physicians and hospital in leadership and management of the integrated entity<br>◆ Recruitment plan, including anticipated changes in the mix of services or specialties |
| Financial management | ◆ Expected financial performance of the physician enterprise<br>◆ Access to capital and capital allocation process<br>◆ Financial reporting, such as changes in funds flow that will alter the clinic's bottom line (e.g., overhead allocation, credit for ancillary profitability)<br>◆ Method for determining changes to the physician compensation formula<br>◆ Billing policies and procedures<br>◆ Patient financial assistance program, which may change to match the hospital's program<br>◆ Changes to payer mix |
| Operations | ◆ Use of EHRs and deciding which system (hospital's or practice's) will prevail<br>◆ Conversion of ancillary services to provider-based<br>◆ Corporate compliance and accreditation requirements<br>◆ Clinical quality initiatives<br>◆ Changes to staffing mix as a hospital-based clinic pursuant to accreditation requirements (e.g., certain tasks or procedures done by licensed nursing staff only)<br>◆ Provider work hours and productivity expectations<br>◆ Changes in the peer review process as a hospital-based clinic |

silos, then the opportunity for miscommunication and physician dissatisfaction is rife. Accordingly, overall responsibility for physician acquisitions—from the identification of practices through the on-boarding process—is best assigned to a single individual. Depending on the anticipated volume of practice acquisitions, establishing a position specifically for this purpose may be helpful.

## Anticipate Medical Staff Reaction

In the absence of a clearly defined and properly communicated physician strategy, hospital executives often encounter animosity from the independent members of the medical staff, who may perceive that the hospital is now competing with them. They may also perceive that limited hospital resources will be shifted away from hospital operations to focus on the development of the employed physician group. These perceptions can create an uncomfortable divide between the employed physicians and the other medical staff. In an effort to appease the independent physicians, the hospital may be tempted to respond by acquiescing to their demands, sometimes at the expense of the employed physicians. For example, the hospital may cancel plans that newly employed physicians had to recruit in a given specialty, if such recruitment might antagonize independent medical staff members in that specialty. Hospitals may also look for creative ways to shift money to the independent physicians via granting directorships, creating leadership roles, or paying for call coverage. While shifting funds may have a short-term benefit, it sets precedents that are very costly not only financially but also with respect to the relationship between the hospital and its physicians, both independent and employed.

Hospital leadership should also be prepared to deal with negative behaviors that independent medical staff members sometimes exhibit when they are poorly prepared for the introduction of employed physicians. For example, independent physicians commonly divert poorly insured or uninsured patients to the employed medical group. In extreme cases, independent physicians are openly hostile to the employed physicians, eventually driving them out of business by spreading false rumors or shutting them out of the call schedule. To ward off this type of reaction, hospitals must gain the support of the medical staff leadership by including them early in the pre-acquisition planning and by creating a forum for them to voice their concerns appropriately.

## NOT JUST A HOSPITAL ANYMORE

For many hospital executives, the prospect of employing physicians is little more than a necessary evil, but one that involves a lot of hard work, a substantial investment, the surrender of control, and potentially significant financial losses. If the undertaking is less than fully embraced, then these fears are likely to become a reality. However, if it is approached with a well-thought-out plan and within the context of an integrated system rather than a hospital-dominated system, the prospects for realizing the benefits of integration are strong. In the post-reform world, if integration is done correctly, hospitals and physicians can achieve together what they cannot accomplish separately, and everyone, including the broader community, will benefit.

Having this mind-set makes all the difference between a true hospital–physician partnership and an environment in which the physicians are dissatisfied, not engaged, and only too willing to share their woes with other physicians in the community. The remainder of this book describes in greater detail the key areas that need to be addressed to create this partnership.

# CHAPTER 2

# Managing the Transaction

*Scott F. Burns, Sean T. Hartzell, and Adam J. Klein*

A SUCCESSFUL AND sustainable physician practice acquisition requires a respect for cultural differences, as well as a clear vision of the ultimate relationship and the expertise to make the changes necessary for realizing this vision. Once a hospital and physician practice have initiated discussions about a potential acquisition, the process should be carefully managed to increase the potential for a successful outcome. Although both parties will participate in the process, the acquiring organization needs to take the lead on the various components of the transaction while allowing the acquired entity to help determine and craft the final outcome.

This chapter will cover the key considerations in acquiring physician practices and employing physicians. Along with the technical components of a transaction, the following key factors for a timely and successful outcome will be discussed:

- Testing the feasibility of a transaction
- Designing and documenting the transaction
- Transition planning
- Getting it right

## TESTING THE FEASIBILITY OF A TRANSACTION

The hospital and physicians should first discuss independently, and then together, what they hope to achieve through integration. In most cases, the hospital can easily articulate what alignment with physicians would mean for it; the greater challenge is to retain flexibility in considering different ways to reach its goals. The physicians, however, often have considerable diversity of opinion as to both how affiliation should be structured and what benefits are expected. The physicians should take the time to discuss these differences, because discussion will help them determine which goals are most important and ultimately move the group toward consensus.

After the objectives of both the hospital and the physicians have been clearly articulated, the parties should take time to understand each other's motivating factors and goals, which will include not only financial arrangements but also strategic, operational, and cultural concerns. The hospital needs to know that the members of physician leadership who engage in this dialogue adequately represent all of the physicians in the group. To that end, the hospital should ensure that the physician group develops an internal communication plan to keep its members informed—not so that the hospital can control this plan, but rather because some physician groups are notoriously poor communicators or include physicians who have diverse agendas.

Once a good fit exists between the parties, the basic feasibility of the transaction needs to be assessed. Sound business planning principles should not be abandoned under pressure to acquire physicians based on strategic goals. Otherwise, hospital managers may consider an acquisition that doesn't go through as a failure but view buying the group as a success even if it means losing money at an unsustainable rate. All too often, buyers will rationalize an acquisition with fanciful claims of "synergies" when, in reality, the arrangement clearly cannot stand on its own merits.

The financial implications of the proposed relationship are of course a critical component of feasibility, and financial projections should be based on realistic assumptions. In most cases, physician productivity will decrease, overhead costs will go up, and the payer mix will shift toward poorly insured and uninsured patients (see Chapter 1). Useful financial analyses include assessments of the net operating income of the post-transaction enterprise, the capital investments that will be required, and the change in hospital operating ratios (e.g., days in cash, collection ratio, revenue and debt) along with the sensitivity of the projections to changes in key assumptions such as number of visits, revenue per visit, and the rate of growth of the provider network.

In addition to financial projections, the proposed relationship should be evaluated on its

+ ability to meet physician objectives,
+ appropriateness to the overall hospital or system strategy,
+ ability to accomplish patient care and clinical program goals, and
+ likelihood of successful implementation and operations.

Exhibit 2.1 provides an example of basic feasibility criteria.

**Exhibit 2.1  Acquisition Feasibility Criteria**

| Category | Criteria |
|---|---|
| Financial | ◆ Acceptable internal rate of return (may vary by investment risk category)<br>◆ Limited investment payback period<br>◆ Minimal negative impact on key financial metrics and ratios (capital, liquidity, operating)<br>◆ Beneficial impact on financial debt covenants, borrowing capacity, and credit worthiness within a reasonable time frame<br>◆ Relative size of capital commitments |
| Operational | ◆ Facility capacity and readiness<br>◆ Management capabilities to absorb and integrate the acquisition<br>◆ Compatibility with existing work flows<br>◆ Level of disruption associated with initial and ongoing integration of acquisition |
| Strategic | ◆ Compatibility with health system strategy<br>◆ Improvement in market position<br>◆ Likely competitive response<br>◆ Implications for management, governance, and organizational structure |
| Political | ◆ Medical staff acceptance<br>◆ Board involvement and approval<br>◆ Achievement of cultural fit |

This level of detail in testing feasibility is critical to ensuring that careful analysis, not wishful thinking, forms the foundation of the transaction. To determine objectively whether the transaction should proceed, comparing the merits of the transaction, both quantitative and qualitative, with a set of predefined standards is important. By comparing the transaction to these standards (and having the discipline not to "cook" the assumptions to meet those standards), the acquiring organization can better determine if it wishes to proceed and can identify reasons for moving forward.

## DESIGNING AND DOCUMENTING THE TRANSACTION

Once the feasibility and basic relationships have been determined, working out the specifics of the transaction begins. Regardless of the specific processes used, careful and inclusive management of the transaction process can go a long way toward determining how successful or difficult the eventual relationship will be. The following paragraphs summarize the documents and time required to complete each step.

## Confidentiality Agreement

A confidentiality agreement, also known as a nondisclosure agreement, is a legal contract between the hospital and medical group that outlines confidential material, knowledge, or information that the parties wish to share with one another but to which they wish to restrict access by third parties, such as other hospitals or competing physicians. The parties agree not to disclose information that may be acquired during the discussion and negotiation process and may agree not to reveal even the existence of a potential acquisition. By this time, the sharing of confidential information is expected for the deal to proceed. However, one or both parties are almost always sensitive with regard to disclosing the terms of third-party agreements, as well as the scale of damages to each party in the event of a breach of confidentiality or disclosure. This confidentiality agreement is the initial step, and it is generally completed before any substantive discussion occurs. Boilerplate confidentiality agreements are available that can be easily adapted to meet specific needs. These agreements can generally be finalized within a week.

## Letter of Intent

A letter of intent (LOI), sometimes called a memorandum of understanding, states in general terms that the hospital and medical group intend to complete an acquisition subject to the successful negotiation of the terms and conditions. The LOI should spell out the major deal points that are agreed to in principle—for example, that group assets will be purchased at fair market value, that a competitive physician compensation system will be developed, and that physicians will be included in the governance and management of the program. In many cases, including an expiration date on the LOI is appropriate, both to move the process along and to make it easier for either party to walk away if the arrangement just isn't coming together. The LOI is generally a nonbinding agreement, in that it does not obligate either party to complete the transaction document; however, certain provisions may be enforceable, as described below.

LOIs and confidentiality agreements may also include standstill or no-shop requirements. *Standstill* in this context simply means that the party cannot make material changes, such as major new capital commitments, sale of assets, or modification of the compensation system, while in negotiations. Hospital standstill requirements are usually limited to actions that could affect the subject acquisition, such as new affiliations with other medical groups or purchase of ancillary services that may affect the group.

*No-shop provisions*, sometimes referred to as exclusivity agreements, are becoming more and more common. Such provisions prohibit the medical group from talking to other hospitals about being acquired and can prevent the hospital from discussing merger or affiliation with other medical groups prior to the conclusion of the current negotiations. While groups and hospitals sometimes resist such restrictions, these precautions can be critical to ensuring that both parties are serious about, and committed to, the proposed relationship. In certain instances, groups will conduct simultaneous negotiations with two or more parties and eliminate bidders at each major round. In such cases, exclusivity is not possible, and hospital management needs to consider its participation in these types of auction-like environments.

An LOI can take between two and four weeks to finalize if a moderate to high level of agreement exists between the hospital and medical group from the outset. If the entities have not yet aligned on even the basic components of an agreement, the LOI can take considerably longer.

## Term Sheet

A term sheet is a more specific outline of the material terms and conditions of the proposed agreement regarding all major issues. It guides legal counsel in preparing the proposed definitive agreement. A term sheet skips most of the formalities and lists deal terms in outline or bullet format.

The term sheet is the most important document in the entire negotiating process in that it defines, as completely as possible, how the parties want to structure the deal and operate jointly after completing the transaction. Creating the term sheet takes up most of the time and energy that the transaction demands. Legal advice will be required to resolve some issues, but the principal representatives of the two entities should direct the term sheet's content. A term sheet should address the following elements:

- ◆ Transaction structure
  - − Asset or stock purchase
  - − Assets and liability included and excluded in the transaction

- Process to arrive at a final valuation and payment period, if applicable
- Employment model to be used (see Chapter 4 for details on potential models)
- Physician-employment specifics, such as
  - compensation: initial methodology and process for revising it;
  - other employment issues: benefits, vesting period, handling of past deferred compensation (tax implications), paid time off (PTO) policies, and so forth;
  - term and termination provisions, including potential sanctions and dismissal; and
  - noncompete clauses following termination.
- Governance structure[1]
  - The boundaries of authority of the hospital and medical group, as well as of any board, operating committee, advisory council, or similar structure formed as part of the transaction
  - The rights and obligations of each entity to
    - be informed of decisions of management or other governance bodies;
    - advise decision makers prior to final decisions;
    - approve specific policy or operational decisions; and
    - retain special majority or reserve powers regarding specified actions, possibly including sale of assets, changes to the compensation system, acquisition of other medical groups, and purchase of a new electronic health record (EHR).
- Valuation process, including
  - the valuation methodology to be used;
  - the selection of the valuation firm; and
  - the process for valuation dispute resolution.
- Compensation and benefits for staff, including any employment agreements or severance packages
- Operational issues and responsibilities, such as
  - oversight and determination of budgets;
  - physician administrative support;
  - identification, implementation, and support of EHR and practice management systems;
  - management of physician recruitment and selection;
  - managed care contracting; and
  - employment and termination of physician office and administrative staff.
- Timing and conditions under which either party can terminate the relationship, and provisions for unwinding the relationship, if necessary
- Major transition issues and timing
- Communication plans

Budgets or financial forecasts are not included in the content of the term sheet. The term sheet should address the process for developing and approving budgets, but financial projections themselves are generally not included among the documents that complete the legal portion of the transaction. However, financial projections are an important part of the planning process and should involve both hospital and medical group representatives to ensure that the pro forma financial forecast is realistic and attainable.

The time required to finalize a term sheet varies considerably depending on the size and complexity of the group being acquired. Two months is the bare minimum, while some term sheets take more than six months. The amount of flexibility that exists in designing the relationship depends on the market position of the hospital and medical group. That is, if the market's dominant hospital and medical group are merging, they will have more flexibility in timing and designing the relationship than would a hospital negotiating with a group that has other hospitals seeking to acquire it. Obviously, the parties must do what is necessary to get the deal done, but in many transactions the urgency is more perceived than real. Rushing to finalize a transaction usually results in increased time, cost, and frustration later on, when the newly integrated parties try to make the affiliation work on a day-to-day basis.

## Definitive Agreements

After a detailed term sheet has been prepared, attorneys are asked to develop the necessary legal documents to complete the legal portion of the transaction. Although this task may seem straightforward, a number of documents need to be prepared, reviewed, revised, and signed before the transaction is complete. These documents include, but are not limited to, the following:

- Acquisition agreement (covering governance and operations)
- Asset purchase agreement
- Physician employment agreement
- Fair market value documentation
- Contract assignments
- Bylaws and articles of incorporation for any new physician entity being acquired
- Severance notification for group staff

When these documents are prepared, substantive issues commonly arise that require continuing negotiation to resolve. In addition, a due-diligence review must be completed to determine whether the financial and operational information used to fashion the agreement is accurate. A period of two to three months is typically needed to have documents ready for signature. However, the actual timeline depends on a number of factors.

The scale and scope of due-diligence procedures and the ensuing integration planning can vary widely, depending on the complexity of the transaction. Exhibit 2.2 summarizes the process and time frames for the various steps. In most circumstances, a point person can coordinate and manage the process effectively, orchestrating efforts by both parties' line managers and outside consultants and attorneys, and can complete the process within three months. In larger deals, such as when multiple physician groups are combining into one larger group for acquisition, the increased complexity and need for synchronization may be better addressed by specialized resources, such as a project management office (see "Getting It Right" below).

**Exhibit 2.2  Summary of Documents and Time Frames for Completion**

| Document | Completion Time Frame |
|---|---|
| Confidentiality agreement | 1 week |
| LOI | 2 to 4 weeks |
| Term sheet | 2 to 6 months |
| Definitive agreements | 2 to 3 months |
| Implementation period | 1 to 2 months |
| **Total time from inception to integration** | **6 to 12 months** |

Note: Time frames are subject to material revision, based on issues identified and approvals required from internal and external stakeholders

## TRANSITION PLANNING

Signed documents are a cause for celebration in recognition of the hard work that has been accomplished. However, the newly merged enterprise cannot be fully functional until financial and operational integration is complete, and the transition to integrated operations should be planned well in advance of the transaction's closing. A detailed implementation plan should specify what tasks will be required and who is responsible for completing them. Because line managers from both organizations will likely be involved for the first time in the transaction, the planning should begin by introducing the participants to one another and orienting them on the details of the acquisition. Sample topics in an implementation plan include the following:

- Conversion of the billing system and collection of pre-merger receivables
- Integration of physician operations into the hospital's purchasing system
- Transfer of employees, human resources (HR) administration, and payroll and benefits from the medical group to the hospital or new enterprise
- Integration of accounting (e.g., revised chart of accounts, crosswalk protocols)
- Integration of information technology (IT), including EHR if appropriate
- Changes in third-party payer contracting (e.g., revised rates, changes to tax-payer identification numbers)
- Credentialing by the hospital and payers as required
- Assignment or cancellation of service contracts and leases
- Compliance training

A lot of moving parts are involved in integrating a medical group into a hospital's structure. The parties should mutually decide which efforts are mandatory and which can be deferred and identify how much can realistically be accomplished within the first year of operation. Quickly integrating a medical group into a hospital's operational and governance systems may be appealing for many reasons, but the organization's administrative capability and political will may simply not support full integration in the near term.


## GETTING IT RIGHT

Creating a successful relationship is challenging under the best of circumstances. The following suggestions will help prevent common mistakes.


### Get Organized to Manage the Process

Hospitals and medical groups often want to get a deal signed as soon as possible and figure out the details of the affiliation after the transaction is complete. This approach puts the focus on negotiating the financial aspects of the acquisition and is generally carried out by the entities' principals and legal advisers. However, after completing the deal, the senior administrators who initiated it are rarely involved in resolving the operational relationships and clinical coordination.

Instead of taking the customary route and forming a negotiating committee made up of the leaders of both organizations, the parties should consider using a number of work groups or task forces—with physicians, group managers, and hospital managers represented on each, along with lawyers or consultants as necessary. Depending on the situation, work groups can include the following:

◆ Asset valuation
◆ Physician compensation
◆ Clinical integration
◆ Third-party contracting
◆ Operations (IT, purchasing, facilities, HR)

To minimize arguing over every perceived gain or loss, work groups can be charged with submitting recommendations to the joint decision makers. This process allows for broader participation by physicians and hospital managers, builds shared understanding of issues, and enables the parties to design workable financial, operational, and strategic relationships. Although time consuming, this process is effective in nurturing a shared culture and demonstrating that the principals are serious about integration.

## Determine Whether the Transaction Requires Dedicated Project Management Support

In more complex transactions, or when multiple acquisitions occur simultaneously, the job of coordinating work-group integration-planning activities is shifted from line managers—who are already busy with their regular jobs—to a project management office (PMO), which can better ensure that milestones are met and issues are resolved. A steering committee, composed of the parties' senior representatives, oversees this endeavor and has ultimate responsibility for determining the conduct and direction of the integration process as well as for critical decision making. The PMO is the conduit between the work groups and the steering committee and is responsible for the following:

◆ Work-group coordination, including task completion and interaction among work groups and resources to satisfy all tasks within the transaction timeline. Interfacing with the steering committee on communications and issues resolution is another key responsibility.
◆ Dependency management, or coordination with the work groups when their progress depends on each other's work.

- Issues management, including the identification of time-sensitive matters and incremental resources needed to meet the expectations created by a task plan or timeline.
- Decision support, by drafting and presenting communication reports to the steering committee and work groups on the status of all due-diligence procedures and integration activities.

The need for this level of project support and infrastructure varies, but it is usually appreciated by all parties after complicated deals are closed, and regretted if it is not instituted soon after the confidentiality agreement is accepted and due-diligence procedures are initiated.

## Manage Communications Carefully

A medical group acquisition of any size means that big changes are forthcoming for both the group and the hospital. Helping the stakeholders understand and respond to those changes in a positive way is an important component of the transaction process. A communication plan identifies the timing, messages, and methods to be used with each stakeholder group. A well-designed communication plan will not only inform stakeholders about what is happening but also tell them how they should feel about the impending relationship.

Hospitals are generally familiar with developing communication plans and often have staff to direct the process. When it is about to acquire a group of physicians, the hospital is likely to begin crafting messages to the hospital's stakeholders without regard to the medical group or community constituencies. If the physicians craft different messages or provide different answers to questions posed to hospital and physician leadership, significant problems can result. For this reason, creating a joint communication plan directed at all stakeholders in the proposed transaction is a key to success. The stakeholders include not only the parties involved in the transaction but also payers, suppliers, the media, regulators, and community leaders.

Each of these stakeholders has a legitimate interest in the transaction and can hinder or even prevent it from happening if concerns and interests are not appropriately addressed. The method of communication and the level of detail provided may vary according to the audience, but the communication plan needs to proactively address all likely questions and concerns, while letting the stakeholders know that the initiative is necessary, that it will be good for the integrating organization, that the parties have a clear vision about what the transaction will look like when completed, and that strong and capable leadership is in place to reach the intended goals. These messages need to be repeated before, during, and after an acquisition. A useful way to remember the messages is the "Four Ps" (Exhibit 2.3).

The hospital and medical group should agree on a written communication plan that specifies who will communicate what messages to which stakeholders, as well as the method of communication and the projected timing for each message. Without such a plan in place, rumors, speculation, misinformation, and anxiety are certain to build and make the process significantly more difficult.

## Anticipate Implications of Multiple Group or Multispecialty Transactions

Special consideration needs to be given to situations in which more than one group is being acquired or new groups are being added to an existing employed network. Resistance is likely to be high if physicians perceive that they are being forced into a larger physician structure. Often, acquired groups fear that they will be controlled or will have their control diluted by other physicians, regardless of specialty.

**Exhibit 2.3 The Essential Elements of Communication**

| The Four Ps | Description |
| --- | --- |
| Purpose | Explain why the hospital is undertaking the transaction, what is wrong with the status quo, and how the participants and others will benefit. |
| Picture | Present a shared vision for a truly integrated delivery system. What does it look like? What services, quality measures, shared governance, and management structures will be involved? This vision of where the hospital is heading should include improved patient care and reduced costs as major drivers of the process. |
| Plan | Share enough detail of the agreed-on structure and operations to convey that the parties know how to reach shared goals and have established a clear timeline. What will be done, by whom, and by when to meet the goals of the transaction? The stakeholders need to be confident that the parties can reach the shared vision. |
| Participation | Provide ways that stakeholders can participate in the process to ensure that their concerns and questions are addressed, however basic. Some stakeholders, such as patients of the medical group, may require only an announcement letter that provides an opportunity for questions, while members of the hospital board may be given opportunities to sit in on work-group meetings and to discuss progress and problems during the transaction process. |

For the hospital that is building an integrated network, standardizing governance and operations under a single authority for employed physicians is obviously preferable to having multiple compensation arrangements, operating policies and procedures, recruitment programs, and care management protocols. However, standardization may not be realistic, at least at the outset, so flexibility is required. If the hospital insists on a one-way-fits-all approach to integration, it risks losing the transaction altogether or bringing in a group that is resentful of the hospital and not likely to be a willing partner.

To successfully integrate groups into a larger structure, the hospital must be unwavering in its goal of a unified physician organization while demonstrating flexibility in timing and asking the physicians to provide leadership in the design and implementation of the ultimate model.

## Avoid Overpaying for Assets

In any transaction, the buyer and seller will have different perspectives, and the purchase of a medical group is no exception. Physicians often have unrealistic expectations, and hospitals too often overpay in an effort to complete the deal. In many, if not most, medical group acquisitions, misunderstandings arise about the appropriate price for goodwill or other intangibles. Physicians often believe that a premium should be paid for the business in place, established revenue stream, ancillary business, name, reputation, and other assets. Most often, the value of the practice comes down to the market value of tangible assets, with little or no consideration for goodwill or other intangibles. While not trivial, the amount paid to each physician can be disappointing. To avoid having this issue derail the deal, the parties can jointly select a qualified third-party valuation firm. Although the physicians may still feel disappointed with the outcome, they will be less likely to direct any negative sentiments at the hospital. Ultimately, the selling physicians need to understand that competitive, stable compensation and benefits—rather than a big buyout check—should be the goal.

Another important consideration is the relationship between the transaction price and the physicians' ongoing compensation. These are often viewed as separate when in fact they are interrelated. Depending on the terms of the arrangement and the valuation methodology used, the acquiring organization could be perceived as paying for referrals. Proper coordination between the business valuation and physician compensation planning activities is therefore important. These considerations are discussed in further detail in Chapter 10.

## Ensure the Retention of Physicians and Key Staff

When one hospital purchases another, the retention of newly acquired administrators is seldom a major concern. Managers are frequently paid to leave. In contrast, the value of a medical group is closely tied to the physicians, owners, and lay executives who are employed by the group. To protect these resources, the term sheet should include a condition requiring that a minimum number of physicians (e.g., 80 percent) enter into an employment agreement with the acquiring entity. Further, early in the process, the group's key administrative staff should be included in discussions about their future role in the merged enterprise, including the anticipated job scope, reporting relationships, compensation and benefit details, and availability of a severance agreement. In the absence of this information, key talent may seek employment elsewhere because of the uncertainty of their current position.

## Plan Time for Securing Internal and External Approvals

Effective leadership from both sides is critical during the stage when the organizations seek approval for the transaction from all internal and external stakeholders. Appropriate administrative leadership and legal counsel will need to review the bylaws of both organizations and develop a coordinated approval plan. The steps involved in this plan may include the formal distribution of all definitive agreements, the implementation of shareholder education sessions, the provision of open forums for questions and answers as well as the dissemination of this information to all shareholders, any necessary modifications to bylaws, and any required voting specific to the transaction or bylaw changes. Simultaneous with the internal shareholder approval process, a plan for securing all necessary external approvals should be developed. Depending on the size of the transaction and the potential market shifts that will result from it, a variety of local, state, and national regulatory agencies may need to weigh in and approve the transaction.

Because the internal and external processes can be tedious, the parties may elect to create a separate project plan to determine the lead time required to ensure all necessary stakeholders have approved the transaction.

## THE BOTTOM LINE

An effective affiliation takes a lot of time to build. After a year or more spent completing a transaction, the real work of economic and clinical integration is just beginning. Given the significant cultural differences between hospitals and physicians, attaining alignment is one of the most difficult challenges that either party will ever undertake. Physicians need assurance that the hospital will be a competent and committed employer and business partner, and establishing that credibility requires time. Most hospitals and health systems with substantial, closely aligned physician enterprises have built this trust over the course of many years—in some cases, several decades. Those that have not yet seriously started down this path will need to move more aggressively to prepare for the post-fee-for-service world. Whatever the final details look like, skillful management of the processes involved in completing a transaction is a major factor in ensuring a successful and stable long-term relationship between the hospital and employed physicians.

## NOTE

1. Physicians typically use *governance* in the context of practice-level or service line–level decision making, whereas hospital management typically views governance as the fiduciary and policy-setting responsibilities of the board of directors—clearly different uses of the term.

# CHAPTER 3

# Physician Organization and Leadership

*Kevin J. Duce and Darin E. Libby*

THE GOAL OF hospital–physician alignment is to create a relationship in which both parties work collaboratively and share in the benefits of attaining improved performance. One of the keys to making this concept a reality is creating an organizational structure that engages physicians and establishes shared management of operations. Physicians will not stay invested and engaged in the larger organization if they are treated as rank-and-file employees, nor will compensation incentives alone produce the full range of physician behaviors necessary for success. Physicians need to be given meaningful roles in functions ranging from day-to-day operational decisions to long-term financial and strategic planning. The purpose of this chapter is to describe the organizational, management, and governance models that should be considered for the employed physician group.

For the sake of simplicity, this chapter regularly refers to physicians as being employed. However, the principles discussed apply equally well to models—such as the California medical foundation model and the Texas 501(a) model—in which, because of state corporate-practice-of-medicine laws, physicians are not employees of the health system but instead provide professional services under contract. As a practical matter, however, these models function very much like employment arrangements.

## THE CENTRAL ISSUE: SHARING CONTROL

At the heart of the matter is the need to share control between the health system and physicians and among the physicians themselves. Structuring and managing the employed physician group is a challenge because everyone involved has a strong desire to maintain control. When a health system acquires a physician practice, most of the business risk transfers to the system, whose administrators are likely risk averse by nature. Having assumed that business risk, they would naturally feel a need to exercise control over the physician group in addition to the operations and strategic direction of the rest of the system.

Unfortunately, this need for control often conflicts with an equally deep-rooted need of physicians—their need for autonomy and professional self-determination. Most physicians are trained to think and act independently when providing patient care, and these habits often shape their perspective on administrative matters. Therefore, they will typically be very protective of their autonomy, not only within the physician group but with respect to the health system as well.

To achieve the full benefits of integration, administrators and physicians will need to adopt a very different set of operating activities than they have in the past. Success in a value-based reimbursement environment requires collaboration that is broad in scope, encompassing all inpatient and outpatient care. Addressing this larger scope of activity is difficult even for the most advanced systems and requires a reassessment of long-held assumptions about how the integrated organization should function. Both hospitals and physicians bring critical skills to the relationship, and the structure and leadership of the integrated enterprise will have a major impact on how effectively those skills are put to use.

## ORGANIZATIONAL STRUCTURE

For the health system that seeks to become a truly integrated organization, clear benefits accrue from building a unified physician organization and standardizing governance and operations under a single authority. For example, the hospital wants to avoid

- negotiating separate compensation arrangements with each physician;
- administering operating policies and procedures that vary by clinical section or group;
- setting recruitment needs and making hiring decisions specific to each group; and
- administering redundant care management protocols across the physician enterprise.

Occasionally, a hospital will acquire a large multispecialty organization and achieve consolidation in a single stroke, but such acquisitions are uncommon. In the vast majority of cases, health systems build their employed physician enterprise through a combination of multiple practice acquisitions and the hiring of new physicians just out of training, and then work to unify the organizational structure over time. Physicians who are considering employment arrangements often seek to maintain as much autonomy as possible and to retain compensation arrangements and patient care protocols that are separate from those already in place for other physicians. Therefore, if the hospital starts out by insisting on a one-way-fits-all approach to integration, it risks losing the transaction altogether or bringing in a group that is resentful of the hospital and not likely to be a willing partner. Accordingly, the process of unifying disparate physicians into a cohesive group usually takes many years and may require flexibility in timing and in the design and implementation of the ultimate model. The traditional migration path is depicted in Exhibit 3.1.

On the left side of Exhibit 3.1 are small practices that have little commonality in their operations and finances. Physicians in these different practices may continue to operate from their preexisting clinic locations and may not be professional colleagues who refer patients to one another. Over time, these practices may become more consolidated by specialty or location and may begin to operate out of common facilities. Eventually, the practices begin to resemble a single multispecialty group of physicians who are employed by the health system, as shown on the right side of Exhibit 3.1.

This migration path has traditionally been useful in standardizing operations and administration, making efficient use of shared services, and generating internal referrals. Significant effort is placed in the following activities:

- Employment terms (e.g., term and termination provisions, noncompete agreements, defined roles and responsibilities) are made uniform and documented in a standard employment agreement.

**Exhibit 3.1 Traditional Migration Path to Consolidation**

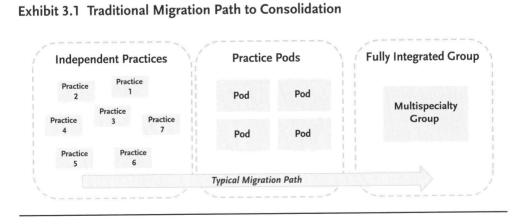

- Compensation arrangements are standardized, with exceptions made to the standard arrangement based on operational and clinical considerations rather than group dynamics and history.
- Back-office billing functions (e.g., claims submission, insurance follow-up, denials management, payment posting) become consolidated under a central billing office, with a standard fee schedule.
- Scheduling, registration, insurance verification, and authorization checking become centralized.
- Information technology and management reporting infrastructure matures, and practice performance begins to be measured against internal and external benchmarks.

This traditional path has several important implications. First, the need for more sophisticated management increases along with the level of complexity. Second, the physicians experience some loss of autonomy and control. However, whether it is a by-product of consolidation or a stated objective, the medical group typically develops a common culture and an identity unto itself. The physicians begin to speak with a more unified voice, which gives them greater clout within the integrated organization. This unity is usually (though not always) considered a desirable outcome, but as the following section observes, it may come at a heavy cost.

## TOO MUCH CONSOLIDATION?

As the physician enterprise begins to represent an employed multispecialty group, the health system may experience an unpleasant and unintended consequence: the physicians may develop a culture and identity that overrides their identification with the health system. If a divide between the physician and hospital components of the organization arises, the two sides may find themselves competing against one another for resources and influence—an actual impediment to integration and alignment. This situation is not necessarily the fault of the physicians; certainly in some instances the hospital, by being overly protective of its prerogatives, bears much culpability for fostering an "us versus them" relationship.

Another unintended consequence is that a unified physician organization can breed divisiveness among the physicians themselves, particularly as value-based reimbursement becomes more prevalent. For example, primary care physicians, who have long felt undervalued and underappreciated for their referrals, may push hard to retain the lion's share of medical management bonuses. Obviously, this tactic does not sit well with specialists, who are accustomed to being the big winners in the income distribution plan.

As a result, some larger and more mature integrated health systems have begun to move away from the multispecialty-group concept by migrating toward a more specialty-based organization, much like the pods shown in Exhibit 3.1. For example, within the context of a multihospital health system, some hospital-based specialties might be consolidated into one physician group that manages services across multiple inpatient facilities, while the breadth of inpatient service offerings is expanded through the creation of new programs, such as surgical hospitalists. This structure reflects the belief that hospital-based specialties are sufficiently different from clinic-based specialties that they merit having a separate structure.

As this book goes to print, the jury is still out on the optimal organizational structure in a value-based reimbursement world. However, the following suggestions should guide future decision making:

◆ The system's strategy should dictate the organization's structure, and a unified medical group construct may not be the best option.
◆ Having a unified, integrated group of employed physicians is not a guarantee of collaborative behavior; integration does not necessarily equate to alignment.
◆ Although moving many disparate physician practices into a more consolidated structure is challenging, reversing course and disaggregating them may be even more difficult. Therefore, having a clear and compelling vision for the integrated physician enterprise before heading down this path is important.
◆ Leaders must determine carefully what the nexus of control should be; that is, how much control resides with the hospital, how much with and among the physicians, and what are the levers that must be pulled effectively in order to ensure success? The answer will vary based on the organization's strategy, the current and future reimbursement environment, and other factors. The organization of the physician enterprise should reflect those considerations and not become an impediment to success.
◆ Regardless of how the physicians are organized, their leaders must be more interested in furthering the strategy of the integrated organization than in supporting the ambitions of the individual physicians.

## PHYSICIAN GOVERNANCE

For the purpose of this chapter, *physician governance* refers to the range of structures and processes by which the employed physician enterprise is directed. These structures and processes go beyond day-to-day management and extend to questions of capital and financial planning, growth, and strategy. Governance structures that include physician participation will vary depending on the specific model that the hospital employs, but each model can accommodate shared responsibility for decisions related to capital and operational budgeting, facility planning, and maintaining accountability for performance. Balancing authority and responsibility is, of course, the major concern in sharing control with physicians.

An effective governance structure gives the group appropriate authority for a clearly defined set of decisions. Hospital and physician leadership should define the authority of the hospital, medical group, and any board, operating committee, advisory council, or similar structure formed as part of the transaction. The parties should then identify the rights and obligations of each to

◆ be informed of decisions of management or other governance bodies;
◆ advise decision makers prior to final decisions;
◆ approve specific policy or operational decisions; and
◆ retain special majority or reserve powers regarding specific actions, e.g., the sale of assets, changes to the compensation system, the acquisition of other medical groups, and the purchase of a new electronic health record (EHR).

The structures for governing the physician enterprise may include any or all of the following:

◆ **Physician cohorts:** Physician cohorts allow physician representation at the specialty or location level, particularly within health systems that do not have a unified physician organizational structure (see Exhibit 3.1). These cohorts may have operational responsibility and authority as defined by the health system, but typically this power is limited in scope. One important function of physician cohorts is that they can provide a means for physicians across multiple employed practices to make their voices heard. Over time, these cohorts can be given greater scope of responsibility to provide standardization across practices.
◆ **Physician council:** Unlike the physician cohorts, the physician council is a governing body that represents the entire physician enterprise. It typically includes 9 to 15 members (the actual number depends on the services, physician makeup, and number of facilities represented), who are elected by the physicians at large. The roles and responsibilities of the physician council may vary but often include the following, subject to the authority delegated to it by the health system:
  – Act as the governing body of the physician enterprise, establishing the overall strategic direction and developing administrative policies and guidelines

- Provide input on the capital and operating budget process
- Maintain accountability for physician enterprise performance
- Oversee quality programs and monitor outcomes metrics
- Review adoption of new technology and procedures
- Oversee physician hiring and termination

Depending on whether a joint operating committee (JOC) is in place (see below), the physician council may include representation from hospital or health system leadership, on either a standing or an ad hoc basis.

- **Joint operating committee:** The JOC includes representatives of both the hospital's or health system's leadership and leaders from the employed physician enterprise. The JOC may exist in conjunction with the physician council or in lieu of it. If both bodies exist, then the physician council often serves as a forum for identifying issues to be brought forward to the JOC, which has greater decision-making authority. In other settings, the physician council and the JOC may be combined into one group.

- **System board:** The system board has ultimate approval authority for the key issues facing the health system, but it typically stays out of day-to-day operational decisions.

Exhibit 3.2 shows a simplified authority matrix for a typical physician enterprise. Although many decisions require both JOC and system board approval (which promotes a true partnership in major decision making), authority is delegated to the greatest extent possible, and the roles of the various entities are clearly defined in advance. The dialogue required to fill out a suitably complex governance matrix is one of the defining events of a successful integration. A useful component of this dialogue is to "stress test" the governance structure by proposing typical events (e.g.,

**Exhibit 3.2 Sample Authority Matrix**

| Function | Physician Cohort | Physician Council | JOC | System Board |
|---|---|---|---|---|
| Budget | Is informed | Advises | Approves | Approves |
| Hiring of new physician (according to established plan) | Approves | Advises | Is informed | Is informed |
| Change in medical group compensation | Advises | Advises | Approves | Approves |
| Selection of EHR (budgeted) | Advises | Advises | Approves | Is informed |

acquiring a new practice, opening or closing a clinic site, developing a capital budget) and talking through how the proposed structure would accommodate these events.

## IMPLEMENTATION OF THE MANAGEMENT STRUCTURE

Consistent with most hospital management structures, leadership of physician practices is often given to a nonclinical administrator—usually an individual with direct management experience in one or more related departments. While this type of management framework is familiar and less complex to implement, the interdisciplinary nature of physician operations and the focus on physician alignment to drive clinical improvements warrant consideration of physician-directed or shared-management (dyad) models. These alternative approaches to leadership composition are shown in Exhibit 3.3.

### Administrator-Led Management

The administrator-led structure places management responsibilities in the hands of a nonphysician leader and has traditionally been the most frequently used model. The benefit of this model is that an experienced administrator possesses the business skills, and likely the operational experience in select departments, to lead the physician organization effectively. The challenge for the administrator, however, is that not having direct patient care responsibilities means she must delegate oversight of and leadership for patient and quality functions. Because physicians are not involved, this model is best utilized as an interim management model when a new group is forming and no recognized physician leader exists. As the physician enterprise begins to consolidate, the need for physician leadership becomes more important.

### Physician-Directed Management

Strong physician organizations often place physicians in meaningful management positions to unify the physicians and enhance hospital–physician alignment. Of all potential leaders, a physician may be best prepared to ensure quality and safety, achieve pay-for-performance (P4P) goals, pursue service development opportunities, and foster relationships with the employed physicians and independent medical staff members. The challenge, of course, is finding physician leaders who

## Exhibit 3.3 Alternative Management Structures

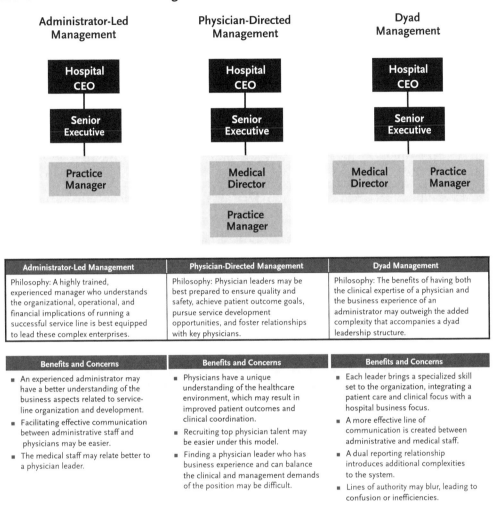

Administrator-Led Management / Physician-Directed Management / Dyad Management

| Administrator-Led Management | Physician-Directed Management | Dyad Management |
|---|---|---|
| Philosophy: A highly trained, experienced manager who understands the organizational, operational, and financial implications of running a successful service line is best equipped to lead these complex enterprises. | Philosophy: Physician leaders may be best prepared to ensure quality and safety, achieve patient outcome goals, pursue service development opportunities, and foster relationships with key physicians. | Philosophy: The benefits of having both the clinical expertise of a physician and the business experience of an administrator may outweigh the added complexity that accompanies a dyad leadership structure. |

| Benefits and Concerns | Benefits and Concerns | Benefits and Concerns |
|---|---|---|
| ■ An experienced administrator may have a better understanding of the business aspects related to service-line organization and development.<br>■ Facilitating effective communication between administrative staff and physicians may be easier.<br>■ The medical staff may relate better to a physician leader. | ■ Physicians have a unique understanding of the healthcare environment, which may result in improved patient outcomes and clinical coordination.<br>■ Recruiting top physician talent may be easier under this model.<br>■ Finding a physician leader who has business experience and can balance the clinical and management demands of the position may be difficult. | ■ Each leader brings a specialized skill set to the organization, integrating a patient care and clinical focus with a hospital business focus.<br>■ A more effective line of communication is created between administrative and medical staff.<br>■ A dual reporting relationship introduces additional complexities to the system.<br>■ Lines of authority may blur, leading to confusion or inefficiencies. |

have the skills, temperament, and time to succeed in this role. Running a complex physician enterprise requires a strong business background and, often, a great deal of patience to function within a highly bureaucratic health system. It also requires a great deal of time, and therefore physician leaders in this model typically do not maintain a clinical practice.

## Dyad Management

In recent years, health systems with more developed physician operations have begun to favor shared management (dyad) structures, which pair a physician with an administrative leader. This construct directly engages physicians in the management of the integrated physician enterprise—one of the key goals of better-performing hospitals. The dyad management model is powerful because it elevates the role of the physician and incorporates clinical insight to better support management decisions. Dyad management structures can be deployed at the enterprise level (to allow the leaders to coordinate on development and clinical integration of the physician enterprise, for example) or at the practice level (to manage day-to-day operations of the practice).

The dyad model combines aspects of the administrator-led and physician-directed models, pairing an administrator and physician to work in tandem to lead the physician enterprise. Ideally, the physician still maintains an active clinical practice in addition to his administrative responsibilities. This structure offers the benefits of both the physician's clinical expertise and the administrator's business experience. Also, it may create a more effective line of communication among administrative, medical, and nursing staff. However, a degree of added complexity accompanies a dyad leadership structure if the roles and responsibilities of the physician and the administrator are not clearly defined. To ensure success, organizations should complete a skills assessment to determine the strengths of each leader. Job descriptions should be clearly defined and should document the span of control and authority of each position. Finally, reporting relationships must be defined and communicated to staff and physicians. Exhibit 3.4 illustrates a division of responsibilities between the dyad leaders.

Although management structures are often illustrated as sets of linked boxes, in reality the boxes contain human beings with strengths, weaknesses, and personalities that should be considered when determining fit for the management construct. Evaluation of alternative management approaches should assess the benefits and drawbacks of the options and implement structures that align with both the strategic goals of the organization and the available leadership talents. Each model has its advantages and disadvantages; however, better-performing organizations most commonly use dyad management structures to balance administrative and clinical leadership in the management of the organization. Transitioning from an administrator-led to a physician-directed or dyad management model requires the development of strong physician leadership, which is essential to creating meaningful integration.

## PHYSICIAN LEADERSHIP DEVELOPMENT

Physician enterprise development demands tight alignment of physician and hospital interests. Regardless of the structures they use to align with physicians, suc-

**Exhibit 3.4  Dyad Leadership Responsibilities**

Physician Leader        Administrative Leader

- Quality of care
- Coordination of care across specialties and services
- Product standardization, cost containment, resource utilization
- Medical staff development
- Research
- Education

- Program development
- Strategic and business planning
- Physician performance monitoring
- Working with hospital leadership to outline organization-wide strategy

- Resource allocation
- Budgeting and financial oversight
- Performance analysis and monitoring
- Coordination with physician leadership
- Coordination of administrative functions across facilities and locations

cessful integrated organizations recognize the need for strong physician leadership and the importance of granting true clinical and operational power to physician leaders. However, few hospitals have ongoing programs to identify and develop strong physician leaders.

Unfortunately, community hospitals rarely have physician leaders who possess both the interest and the ability to lead an integrated physician enterprise. Appointing the physician with the strongest clinical skills or longest tenure to the leadership position is frequently tempting. However, the skills required to be a strong clinician are different from the skills needed to be a strong physician leader. Often, the hospital has to identify a physician with potential leadership capabilities who has the support of the group and then work with that physician to develop the skills necessary to be an effective leader. If the organization needs to recruit a physician leader from the outside, the existing physicians should be engaged in the process to ensure they support the appointed leader. The existing physicians' approval of the selected candidate is critical.

Physician leaders should be appointed at multiple levels in the organization to ensure the integration of patient care areas throughout the enterprise, as well as to create a pipeline of future leaders. As physicians demonstrate leadership skills at lower levels in the organization, they can expand their roles and take on greater responsibilities at higher levels. Exhibit 3.5 summarizes typical physician leadership responsibilities and required attributes by organizational level.

**Exhibit 3.5  Physician Leadership Levels**

| Level | Responsibilities | Attributes |
|---|---|---|
| Enterprise | ◆ Planning and development<br>◆ Oversight of operations<br>◆ Management of enterprise resources | ◆ Ability to think strategically<br>◆ Ability to understand financial requirements and manage overall budget and resource needs |
| Group | ◆ Oversight of clinical network (e.g., primary care, specialists) | ◆ Ability to represent needs of several specialties<br>◆ Ability to identify recruiting and development needs |
| Service line | ◆ Clinical and administrative coordination between physicians and hospital | ◆ Ability to manage across specialties<br>◆ Ability to balance needs of physicians and the organization |
| Division or department | ◆ Administrative responsibilities for division operations (e.g., scheduling) | ◆ Strong clinical leader<br>◆ Strong organizational skills |

With clinical coordination growing in importance throughout the hospital industry, the shortage of qualified physician leaders is not surprising, but these are the professionals needed to achieve any sustainable progress in reducing costs and improving quality. The search for practitioners who will provide the needed clinical coordination leadership should begin very early in the integration process, whether those physicians and nurses are developed in-house or recruited from outside.

## THE BOTTOM LINE

To be successful, hospitals and physicians will need to work together more closely, and on a broader range of initiatives, than either has in the past. This collaboration requires the development of an integrated physician enterprise that speaks with a unified voice and has the ear of the employing health system. Having appropriate organizational, leadership, and governance structures in place is an essential component for developing these characteristics.

When developing these structures, healthcare leaders should

- continue to push toward a unified physician enterprise, recognizing that this effort will take years to accomplish;
- integrate strong physician leadership at all levels of the organization;
- invest time and effort in defining responsibilities, expectations, and reporting accountabilities for each management position; and
- develop a governance structure that includes physicians and supports clinical integration and alignment across the organization.

# CHAPTER 4

## Developing a Sustainable Physician Compensation Model

*Joshua D. Halverson and James W. Lord*

COMPENSATING PHYSICIANS APPROPRIATELY is one of the most difficult challenges that healthcare leaders will face. Huge sums of money are at stake, solutions are complex to administer, frequent adjustments are necessary, and the process is guaranteed to be politically sensitive and charged with emotion. Even if everything is done right, some stakeholders are sure to be left feeling dissatisfied. It is no wonder, then, that even the mention of a potential change in physician compensation is met with dread, frustration, and, ultimately, avoidance.

Paying physicians used to be straightforward. That is no longer the case, however, and it will only continue to become more complex. In the past, government programs and closed-panel HMOs (e.g., Kaiser Permanente) paid physicians a salary, while the vast majority of physicians were in private practices and paid themselves based on cash receipts less expenses. As an increasing number of physicians migrate into employed medical groups and group practices become larger and more sophisticated, compensation arrangements are becoming more complex.

In most markets, fee-for-service (FFS) remains the dominant form of reimbursement, and therefore productivity usually determines the lion's share of compensation arrangements. However, as the healthcare industry moves inevitably toward more value-based payment methodologies, the financial incentives for an integrated organization will change fundamentally. This change means that the incentives for physicians must also change, because the physicians' activities will make or break the organization under value-based care.

The purpose of this chapter is to describe the essentials of physician compensation. Many of these elements apply whether the health system operates in a traditional FFS system or in a market with more value-based reimbursement. However, given the recent focus on the transition to value-based reimbursement, the chapter specifically addresses this topic as well.

49

# ESSENTIAL CHARACTERISTICS
# OF A PHYSICIAN COMPENSATION PLAN

During the physician acquisition craze of the 1990s, physicians were often placed in salary-based compensation arrangements, with disastrous results. Health systems have learned from this experience and are building incentives into the compensation plan, but the solutions are still less than ideal. Therefore, reviewing some of the essential characteristics that any physician compensation arrangement should have is worthwhile.

◆ **Alignment of incentives:** Perhaps the most important objective, and the most damaging if it is not met, is the need to align the incentives of the physicians and the parent organization—that is, the physicians do well financially when the hospital's objectives are met. If the organization's professional fees are driven by volume, then the physicians should have a meaningful productivity incentive; if capitation, quality, access, or other factors are more meaningful, then the physicians' compensation should reflect those incentives. Keeping these incentives aligned is a challenge when the payer environment is in flux. However, in the absence of any incentives (i.e., salary-based compensation), the employing organization should expect the physicians' efforts to reflect whatever they personally value most.

◆ **Appropriateness of financial incentives:** Leaders should resist the urge to tie financial incentives to every desired physician behavior or to place physicians' pay at risk for things that they cannot directly control. Doing so will create physician dissatisfaction and will bog down the compensation planning process. Leaders should therefore make sure that both the size and the structure of financial incentives are appropriate relative to what the organization is trying to accomplish. In many cases, acceptable results can be achieved simply by providing objective performance feedback, particularly when this feedback is shared with other physicians or if the individual's performance relative to her peers can be demonstrated.

◆ **Market competitiveness:** Obviously, the compensation and benefits package needs to be competitive to recruit and retain quality physicians. The difficulty is that what's competitive is a largely subjective concept and often ill informed. Therefore, reliance on external benchmarks becomes necessary. One of the dangers in benchmarking is that often the default position is to start at median compensation as a minimum expectation, and then layer on incentives to allow physicians to exceed the median with relative ease. By definition, however, fully half of all physicians earn below the median, so below-median compensation does not necessarily mean below-market compensation.

◆ **Flexibility:** Compensation planning is a journey, not a destination. Circumstances are constantly shifting, requiring adjustments to the compensation model. In particular, the shift from volume- to value-based reimbursement will require changes in the way physicians are paid. Therefore, anticipating these changes and building flexibility into the model to accommodate them is helpful. For example, if sizable pay-for-performance (P4P) quality incentives are anticipated in the future, organizations should consider including a very modest incentive for the physicians now and expanding it over time. Setting this expectation up front will reduce the need for a major redesign later.

◆ **Transparency:** Metrics and incentives should be easy for physicians to understand. Yet, physicians often have difficulty understanding how their compensation arrangement works. The more complicated the compensation arrangement is, the greater this difficulty will be—and the greater the difficulty in administering it properly. Compensation arrangements should also be accompanied by scorecards to provide physicians with useful information regarding how they are performing relative to incentives and how their pay is calculated—something that most organizations do not do effectively.

◆ **Consistency:** Whenever possible, the compensation model should be applicable across specialties and service sites. Such a model is not always feasible, and usually some specialties will be paid on a separate plan. However, developing consistency will not only minimize the already substantial administrative burden but also avert some of the dissatisfaction that inevitably arises when physicians perceive that their compensation arrangement is the least favorable of the bunch. At a minimum, the plans across specialties should align with the same system goals.

◆ **Acceptance by physicians:** No compensation arrangement will be embraced enthusiastically by every physician in the organization. However, if the majority of physicians do not view the compensation arrangement as fundamentally equitable and reasonable, their objections must be addressed through better communication or a redesign of the plan.

## COMPENSATION FUNDS FLOW

The funds flow relating to physician compensation must be well understood and properly designed. This process begins with payer contracting and reimbursement for physician and related services. The compensation plan itself consists of compensation funding—the methodology for making a pool of compensation funds available for the physicians in aggregate—and the distribution of those funds to the individual physicians. All of these elements need to be structured so that they produce incentives that are consistent and aligned. These relationships are shown in Exhibit 4.1.

## Contracting and Reimbursement

Alignment of the physician compensation plan with the incentives of the organization begins with the organization's overall objectives, which should translate to a cogent strategy for contracting with payers. The contracting function will determine reimbursement and should be supported by the physician compensation funding and distribution plans.

Accordingly, the contracting strategy should answer the following specific questions:

◆ How aggressively should the organization pursue value- and population-based contracts? Which value-based methodologies are most appropriate to the organization's situation and capabilities? Is full-risk contracting a viable option?

**Exhibit 4.1 Typical Funds Flow**

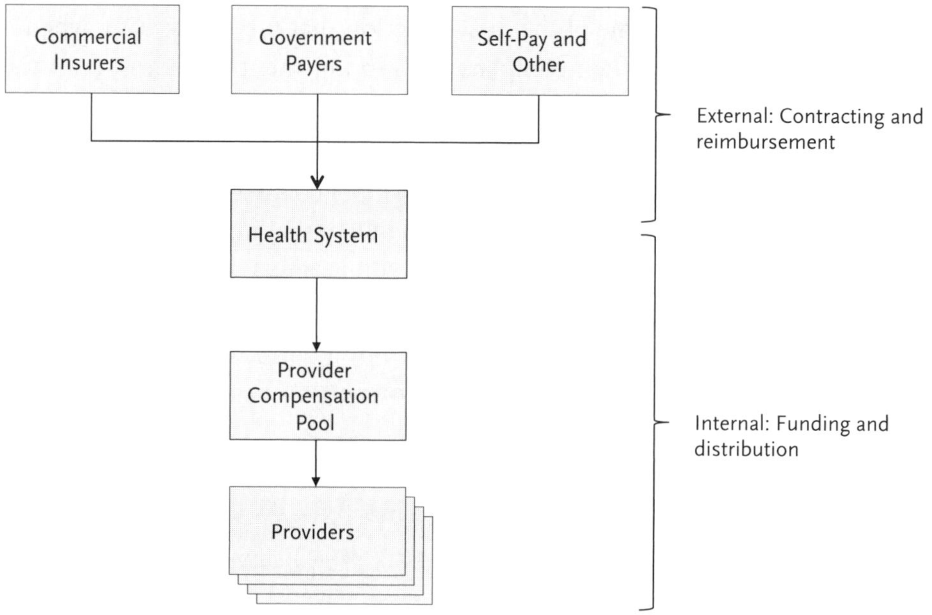

- Are there opportunities to partner with area employers in value-enhancing initiatives?
- Will the organization's priority be a Medicare strategy, a commercial payer strategy, or a balance of the two?
- Are inpatient contracting and ambulatory contracting appropriately coordinated, and does the organization have adequate information on the yields associated with existing ambulatory contracting?
- How well do the revenue cycle functions perform? Do billing and collections issues need to be addressed?

The answers to these questions will have a major influence on how physician compensation is structured. They also require an understanding of internal organizational capabilities, the local hospital and physician market, and the local payer market. Administrators may not be well versed in all of these areas and may therefore want to meet with payers to gain a different perspective. Additional information on payer contracting is provided in Chapter 11.

## Funding and Distribution

In the funding step, the compensation pool is first established according to a defined set of rules that support the overall goals of the system. These funds are then distributed to individual physicians following a second set of rules, which are usually similar but not identical to the rules used to create the pool. For example, the pool may be funded using a blended compensation per work relative value unit (RVU) amount but distributed partly on an equal-share basis and partly on an individual productivity basis, using specialty-specific compensation per work RVU values. The implication is that physicians' individual compensation is determined by the performance of their peers as well as their own individual performance. If the physicians are then allowed some latitude in deciding on the distribution formula, the compensation plan can serve as an excellent way to promote a common group culture. Few tasks are more difficult than determining how to distribute compensation funds, but allowing physicians to take ownership of this process will help build a stronger group.

Finally, the compensation pool that has been established through the funding process is distributed to the individual physicians in the group. Ideally, the physicians will decide on a distribution methodology that aligns with the funding methodology and thus encourages the individual physicians to exhibit those behaviors that will result in maximum funding to the group. This alignment of funding and distribution makes it all the more important for the funding methodology to be consistent with the system's objectives.

In systems where the physicians are not employed but serve under a professional services agreement (PSA), having separate funding and distribution steps is the preferred methodology for paying the physicians. The health system funds the independent medical group according to the formula described in the PSA, and then the physicians distribute those funds as they see fit.

In some systems, the funding and distribution functions are combined into one—each physician's compensation is determined by his individual performance and is not affected by the performance of other physicians in the group. The physicians do not participate in a pool per se; rather, total physician compensation is simply the aggregate of each physician's independently calculated compensation. This methodology is usually less confusing to the physicians and easier for them to accept, particularly if they have a history of being employed. However, by taking the group out of the equation, this model represents a missed opportunity to build a common group culture.

## Physician Involvement in Compensation and Contracting Oversight

Given the close relationship between the contracting and compensation functions as well as the central role of physicians, engaging physician leaders is critical to identify areas for clinical value improvement that can be used to negotiate better payer contracts (higher rates or more favorable terms) and physician compensation. Linking these clinical initiatives to P4P, and ultimately to risk, is crucial for a successful transition to a value-based environment. Hospital-owned physician groups are too often viewed as a department of the hospital, where physicians are managed much like other hospital employees. The hospital's contracting staff and human resources (HR) leadership are often very protective of their prerogatives and processes, seeing no need to share authority or be accountable to physician employees. However, if employed physicians are to be true partners in the growth of the enterprise as a whole, they must have leadership roles in contracting and compensation.

Enterprise-wide clinical leadership, contracting, and compensation committees are structures that effectively ensure input from all stakeholders, including physicians. In addition to allowing physicians to serve in decision-sharing roles (as opposed to mere advisory roles), these structures acknowledge that physicians do much of the heavy lifting required to improve both quality and efficiency. Physician activities include but are not limited to the following:

- Determining and implementing new clinical standards
- Improving electronic health record (EHR) systems to support population health management
- Navigating and reconstructing operational processes to support the coordination of patient care
- Sharing data with peers to identify variation and opportunities for improvement

Given their central role in improving quality and efficiency, physicians must be engaged in both the strategic and tactical components of payer contracting and also must understand the implications of contracting initiatives for physician compensation.

## COMPENSATION DESIGN AND REDESIGN PROCESS

The compensation design and redesign process is critical for developing a sound compensation plan and achieving physician buy-in, yet the importance of the process is frequently underestimated. Establishing a compensation committee consisting of both administrators and physicians to oversee the process is advisable. The physicians on the committee should be thought leaders who are well respected and trusted to act with impartiality.

Successful compensation design and redesign approaches generally include three sequential stages:

1. **Assessment:** The purpose of the assessment phase is to establish a baseline understanding of the existing compensation arrangement's strengths and weaknesses. This assessment is necessary because the various stakeholders in the plan will invariably have differences of opinion. While the assessment may not result in complete consensus regarding the plan, it will at least serve to identify where opinions differ and should create more realistic expectations about the outcome of the process. Key activities include
   - gathering internal data on past compensation and productivity;
   - interviewing physicians about expectations and preferences;
   - conducting external benchmarking by specialty and geography; and
   - identifying issues with the existing compensation plan that must be addressed during the redesign.
2. **Design:** In the design phase, various conceptual models are vetted by the compensation committee, and then the preferred model is tested using the

group's actual historical data as inputs. This testing is an iterative process that involves examining the outputs of the model and adjusting the variables until the desired results are achieved. Specific activities include

- developing consensus regarding principles of the compensation plan;
- identifying options and a preferred conceptual model;
- developing a financial model, including (1) quantifying the variables, (2) creating financial projections, and (3) revising the model as required based on the results;
- addressing additional considerations that fall outside of the basic conceptual model (see "The Devil Is in the Details" box); and
- communicating the proposed plan to the physicians at large.

3. **Implementation:** Implementation consists of creating the infrastructure for administering the compensation plan on an ongoing basis. Whereas the design phase is more conceptual in nature, the implementation phase addresses a myriad of details regarding how the plan will work in practice, including

- special policies for part-time or shared-practice physicians;
- measurement period for productivity and other incentive variables (e.g., monthly versus quarterly, date of service versus date of posting, use of continuous rolling averages versus periodic reconciliation); and
- frequency of incentive payments.

All of these details must be documented, and the necessary tools and processes to administer the plan must also be developed. In some cases, providing a side-by-side comparison of the old and new models for a period of time—before implementing the new model, after, or both—allows physicians to gain an appreciation of how the new plan affects them.

## COMPENSATION FOR NEWLY INTEGRATED PHYSICIANS

When new physicians are brought into an employed physician group, initial compensation is sometimes determined during the negotiating process rather than through a more thoughtful redesign process as described above. Such one-off compensation arrangements are particularly the case when an existing arrangement is not already in place and time is of the essence. In this situation, the acquiring entity should establish up front that an interim compensation methodology will be used immediately after the close of the transaction but that soon thereafter a compensation redesign will occur. Naturally, the physicians will want to negotiate as much protection for themselves in the new plan as possible.

### The Devil Is in the Details

Here are some of the many questions that need to be answered before a compensation plan can be successfully implemented:

- **Ancillary or outside revenue:** How will ancillary or outside revenue be allocated among group members (e.g., equal shares, based on use, based on ownership)?

- **Capitation revenue:** How is capitation revenue distributed among the group? What is the weight of incentives for productivity versus efficiency?

- **Part-time providers:** How does the plan handle part-time providers? Is their productivity normalized?

- **Shared practices:** Do physicians in a shared practice share the compensation, or is each treated as a part-time physician?

- **Advanced practice clinician productivity:** Does APC productivity count toward a supervising physician's productivity?

- **New physicians:** Will the group provide income guarantees? If so, for how long?

- **Work standards:** How many clinical hours per week are required for full-time providers?

- **Plan draws and reconciliations:** Over what period does the plan draw from, and when is the draw reconciled with actual productivity?

- **Nonclinical duties:** How will physicians be compensated for nonclinical duties (e.g., practice management responsibilities, outreach staffing, research)?

- **Expense management:** How will physicians be incentivized to manage expenses in their clinic?

Because the newly acquired physicians are sure to have a very different perspective than the acquiring entity, the hospital often must make them understand certain unanticipated impacts and implications, including the following:

- **Higher benefit costs:** The hospital benefit package is often more robust and costly than private practice benefits, and this higher cost contributes significantly to deficits for new practices. Although many physicians are keenly attuned to the deficits, the benefit package is often not perceived as better by physicians or their staff.

◆ **Paid time off (PTO):** When physicians are paid according to productivity, PTO is frequently confusing to both the physician and the hospital HR staff. If the physician is not paid when he doesn't work, PTO becomes *allowable* time off, not *paid* time off.

◆ **Revenue recognition:** In most hospital-based systems, accrual accounting replaces cash accounting when revenue is calculated. If physician compensation is based on revenue, the use of a uniform discount rate can significantly affect compensation and be difficult to explain to physicians who have a beneficial mix of patients.

◆ **Perceived equity:** When physicians have been brought in to the group at different times from different specialties, differences in compensation methodologies inevitably exist. Many specialties present unique compensation challenges that prevent a single plan from applying to all physicians. Examples include specialties that have significant ancillary revenue, such as oncology and cardiology; specialties that have historically had equal compensation, such as radiology; and hospital-based specialties, including emergency medicine and hospitalists.

◆ **Administrative requirements:** Hospitals are frequently not prepared for the reality that compensation will be an ongoing part of their relationship with physicians and that it will require significant staff resources to be appropriately administered, monitored, and periodically revised.

## COMPENSATING PHYSICIANS FOR THE SUPERVISION OF ADVANCED PRACTICE CLINICIANS

The increasing reliance on advanced practice clinicians (APCs), also known as midlevel providers or allied health professionals, is an ongoing phenomenon that will likely continue into the foreseeable future. APCs present an interesting challenge to physician compensation because they are resources that generate both revenue and expenses under the supervision of physicians, and as such they have a major impact on physicians' personal productivity and overall practice economics. Accordingly, creating appropriate compensation structures for both the physicians and the APCs is necessary.

Addressing compensation for APCs should begin by understanding the role of the APC within the practice, because this role can vary significantly (Exhibit 4.2).

At one end of the spectrum, the APC is an extension of the physician's practice and takes over routine functions for the physician. At the other end of the spectrum are APCs who function essentially as independent practitioners, with limited oversight from the physician.

The APC's role has important implications for compensation. To the extent that she serves as a physician extender, the APC generates little revenue directly but may contribute significantly to the physician's productivity (whether measured as work RVUs, collections, capitated panel size, and so forth). The physician directly influences the activities of the APC, and therefore the APC is typically paid on a salary-based model. Any productivity generated by the APC is generally awarded to the physician. To ensure that the APC is utilized appropriately, the cost of the APC should be allocated back to the physician via the compensation model. Otherwise, the health system effectively pays for the APC twice—once for the APC's actual salary and benefits and again through the incremental physician productivity that the APC makes possible—and conflicts over APC staffing and compensation levels are likely to arise.

To the extent that the APC is an independent practitioner, she should be compensated much like physicians, with personal incentives for work RVUs, maintenance of patient panels, and so forth. However, because APCs usually operate in team-based practices with multiple providers, paying them a significant base salary is usually the best way to avoid unintended competition among providers. Although these APCs may require only minimal physician supervision, providing the physicians with a stipend or gain-sharing compensation element for their oversight may be necessary.

**Exhibit 4.2 APC Scope-of-Practice Spectrum**

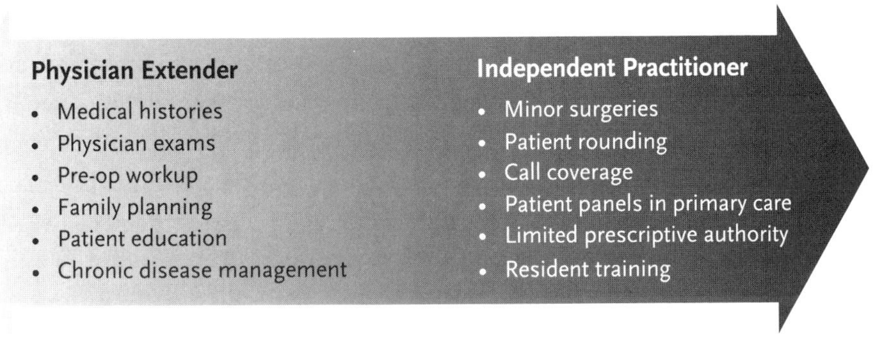

**Physician Extender**
- Medical histories
- Physician exams
- Pre-op workup
- Family planning
- Patient education
- Chronic disease management

**Independent Practitioner**
- Minor surgeries
- Patient rounding
- Call coverage
- Patient panels in primary care
- Limited prescriptive authority
- Resident training

# FEE-FOR-SERVICE REIMBURSEMENT: VOLUME-BASED COMPENSATION

As medical groups have increased in size and hospitals have employed more physicians, compensation arrangements have grown in variety and complexity. Still, productivity-based models remain the dominant form of compensation for now and therefore deserve mention. Productivity variables that can be used in compensation calculations are shown in Exhibit 4.3. In recent years, the work RVU has emerged as the basis for a majority of employed physician compensation arrangements because it is payer blind, it is a reasonable proxy for physician work effort, it is relatively easy to administer, and industry benchmarks are readily available.

### Exhibit 4.3 Volume-Based Compensation Variables

| Variable | Advantages | Disadvantages |
|---|---|---|
| Work RVUs | ◆ Most accepted measure of physician effort<br>◆ Payer blind<br>◆ Consistent comparison of physician productivity | ◆ May not reflect cash received in the practice<br>◆ Difficult to understand derivation |
| Collections | ◆ Direct measure of cash inflow<br>◆ Aligned with reimbursement | ◆ Affected by payer mix and effectiveness of billing and collections<br>◆ Uses cash accounting rather than accrual accounting |
| Gross charges | ◆ Aligned with FFS<br>◆ Payer blind | ◆ Influenced by fee schedules<br>◆ May not reflect productivity or actual reimbursement |
| Visits | ◆ Easily measurable and understandable | ◆ Not meaningful for procedural specialties<br>◆ Does not consider acuity or length of visit<br>◆ Not aligned with financial strategy |
| Panel size | ◆ Appropriate for large capitated panels or patient-centered medical home<br>◆ Improves accessibility | ◆ Lack of accepted benchmarks<br>◆ Requires age, sex, and acuity adjustments |

# PHYSICIAN COMPENSATION IN
# A VALUE-BASED REIMBURSEMENT ENVIRONMENT

Although the dominant compensation models today are productivity based, their prevalence is changing as both public and private sector initiatives point to the reimbursement of providers based on the efficiency and effectiveness of care rather than the volume of services. A variety of new contracting models are emerging, discussed in some depth in Chapter 11. These types of arrangements, albeit small in initial scope, are driving changes in delivery, such as patient-centered medical home (PCMH) models that necessitate more team-based care. As a result, most organizations are considering a broader array of compensation incentives that balance the continued need for productivity with rewards for efficient clinical outcomes.

## The Challenge of Tying Compensation to Value-Based Reimbursement

Under many value-based payment methodologies, such as P4P, bundled payments, and shared savings plans, the financial incentives emphasize different activities and results, and the link between the financial reward and physician activities is less direct. In the FFS world, this is a nonissue because the cause-and-effect relationship is very clear: If the goal is to maximize revenue, then incentivizing physicians to be more productive is easy. With value-based reimbursement, which structures incentives around principles such as quality and efficiency, the organization's financial incentive may not translate as directly to specific physician behaviors that can be rewarded via the compensation plan.

Largely because of this challenge, some organizations are reaching the conclusion that salary-based models are the only workable solution in this environment. The reasoning is that the multitude of desired physician behaviors is too complex to measure in a meaningful way and that paying for a subset of behaviors while ignoring others will ultimately be counterproductive. However, as noted earlier in this chapter, in the absence of economic incentives or a strong group culture, physicians will naturally do the things that they personally value most. Few organizations have a strong enough culture to allow salary-based models to work successfully, and those that do all developed that culture over many years. However, even large, established systems that have traditionally paid a flat salary, such as Kaiser, are moving toward increasing levels of variable incentives as part of their physician compensation plans. Incorporating such variable incentives allows them to provide a more balanced approach to reward high performers and promote access.

Structuring compensation arrangements in a value-based environment requires careful determination of the specific physician behaviors that will lead to favorable results for the health system, as well as deciding how best to incentivize those behaviors, both in aggregate (i.e., compensation funding) and at the individual level (i.e., compensation distribution). This kind of structure is likely to involve payment based on some combination of leading indicators (i.e., if we pay physicians to do X, we hope that will result in outcome Y) and lagging indicators (i.e., if we share the financial rewards of outcome Y with physicians, we hope they will figure out what X needs to be and will do that). Note that the word *hope* occurs in both scenarios because there will always be some uncertainty that the incentive will produce the desired outcome. Several potential performance metrics can be incorporated into the incentive plan (Exhibit 4.4).

Another challenge in tying physician compensation to value is the highly sophisticated administrative infrastructure needed to pull it off. Whereas productivity data are easily pulled from the practice management system, the metrics for cost and quality involve a much greater investment, including access to clinical data via the EHR, sophisticated data analysis and reporting, and staff to provide quality and resource management. Even with this investment, the output will be less than perfect, so the system and the physicians will need to learn how to work with information that is "good enough."

## Distributing Capitated Dollars

For groups that receive a per member per month (PMPM) payment for their services, distributing those dollars internally presents a particular challenge. Ironically, some groups that accept capitation continue to pay themselves based on productivity, reasoning that this method represents the fairest distribution of those dollars even though it creates incentives that run counter to the incentives of capitation. Particularly when the patient population is mixed (both managed care and FFS), groups may determine that they cannot and should not treat patients differently based on reimbursement, and that until capitation becomes the dominant form of reimbursement, they will stick with their traditional, productivity-based model.

On the other hand, for groups that are predominantly capitated or have greater experience with capitation, payment based on panel size is the more common and preferred means of distributing capitated dollars. Whereas, in the FFS environment, individual physicians have a great deal of flexibility to build their practices independently, the number of capitated lives is determined by arrangements made between the employing organization and the payer. Therefore, it becomes

## Exhibit 4.4 Value-Based Performance Metrics

| Goal | Incentive | Performance Metric |
|------|-----------|--------------------|
| Reward a high level of clinical activity that will result in increased revenues and improved patient access | Work effort | ◆ Panel size<br>◆ Office hours or availability |
| Encourage cost-effective and clinically appropriate care | Medical management and quality | ◆ Healthcare Effectiveness Data and Information Set (HEDIS) indicators<br>◆ Adherence to clinical protocols<br>◆ Inpatient days per 1,000 population<br>◆ Ambulatory visits per 1,000 population<br>◆ Selective utilization rates (e.g., emergency department visits, MRIs)<br>◆ Readmission rates |
| Acknowledge a patient-oriented focus and the importance of patient satisfaction to enrollment growth | Patient satisfaction | ◆ Patient satisfaction surveys<br>◆ Patient complaints and compliments and panel retention |
| Reward the performance of nonclinical activities that benefit the organization | Group citizenship | ◆ Committee participation<br>◆ Peer review<br>◆ Specific work-group outcomes<br>◆ Staff surveys |

incumbent on the employing organization to ensure that the size of the physician workforce aligns with the number of lives being contracted for.

Another concern is that physicians with an adverse patient mix in their panel will have to expend more time and effort caring for these patients, and therefore some sort of normalizing adjustment is desirable. Most organizations do not have the wherewithal to adjust for adverse patient mix; however, for those that do, a good practice is to make adjustments based on the risk adjustment factor scores or hierarchical condition categories of the patients within that panel. Also, holding individual physicians at risk for managing the cost of care of their own patients is generally not reasonable; rather, managing costs is a function of the utilization management team, with risk being borne at the organizational level.

## Establishing Fair Market Value

One challenging aspect of paying physicians in a value-based environment is determining fair market value (FMV) compensation. Physicians who are highly successful at managing costs and improving outcomes will be extremely valuable and should be appropriately rewarded for their efforts. As of this writing, little precedent exists for establishing FMV in the new environment, yet of course this does not reduce the need to address FMV. However, as Chapter 10 discusses in detail, that compliance risk can be mitigated by demonstrating that the underlying economics of the arrangement are commercially reasonable—that is, they make sound business sense on their own merits—without taking into account the volume or value of referrals. The following guidelines may help achieve this aim:

- The health system should pay physicians for achieving value-based performance targets only if a tangible economic benefit accrues to the system for attaining those targets.
- The economic benefit of achieving value-based targets should be shared equitably between the physicians and the system.
- Performance incentives should reward genuine improvement, not just uphold the status quo.

Most important, the amount of value-based incentive payments should not drive compensation outside the normal range, regardless of the physicians' level of performance. As financial incentives shift more toward value over volume, a significant redistribution of physician compensation among the different specialties will take place, but this redistribution will play out over a matter of years. Value-based incentive payments should not get so far ahead of the market that physicians are earning at levels that make them outliers.

## Managing the Transition from Volume to Value

Clearly, the changes in reimbursement expected in the coming years will transform how physicians are paid and what they are incentivized to do. This transition represents not only an administrative challenge for organizations but also a complete change in emphasis for physicians, who will be asked to perform new roles and adopt a style of practice for which most of them were not trained. For these reasons, the shift to a compensation plan that is not based on productivity will most likely need to occur over several years (Exhibit 4.5).

**Exhibit 4.5 Sample Transition from Productivity-Based Compensation**

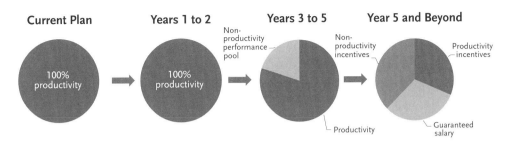

With this transition comes the significant challenge of keeping the incentives of physicians (the compensation plan) aligned with the incentives of the employing organization (payer reimbursement). If the organization moves into value-based physician compensation before securing value-based payer contracts, it risks suffering a drop in productivity and revenue. However, if it moves into P4P or population-based contracts while physicians are paid based on productivity, costs are likely to exceed revenue.

As suggested in the compensation-planning section of this chapter, accompanying this transition with parallel calculations of the pre- and post-implementation plans gives physicians the opportunity to understand and adjust to the new plan before it is fully implemented.

## THE BOTTOM LINE

Physician compensation in an integrated group presents many challenges, but a few core concepts can go a long way toward avoiding conflict and implementing successful compensation plans:

◆ Coordinate physician compensation with the organizational contracting strategy, to ensure that physician compensation incentives are kept in alignment with reimbursement incentives.
◆ Establish explicit processes and principles for determining compensation within the system.
◆ Transition to value-based compensation incrementally.
◆ Understand that compensation systems require periodic enhancements and revisions to remain financially and strategically viable.

# CHAPTER 5

# Optimizing the Physician Enterprise's Operational Performance

*Jennifer K. Gingrass and Michelle L. Holmes*

A CONUNDRUM IN the development of an integrated health system is that creating an effective employed physician group is strategically necessary but financially challenging. Regardless of the size of the group, the typical scenario is that during the assembly of the physicians from independent practices to employment, the group begins to sustain losses that are significantly larger than anticipated. The employing system is then faced with an urgent priority to stop the hemorrhaging of capital while maintaining the momentum of growth. This chapter will discuss the causes of losses, how to set realistic expectations, and the most efficient ways to establish and operate an employed physician group.

## "WE'RE LOSING HOW MUCH?"

A fundamental question in improving financial performance is what, if any, loss is "acceptable"? Stated another way, what are appropriate targets for improvement initiatives? In the early days of hospital employment (late 1980s through mid-1990s), primary care physicians (PCPs) represented the vast majority of employed physicians, and nascent systems were shocked when losses reached $80,000 to $100,000 per physician per year. A best-practice standard was thought, perhaps naively, to be losses averaging under $50,000 per physician per year. After nearly 20 years of growth in employment of physicians by hospitals, no significant progress appears to have been made in improving financial results. In fact, in national surveys health system–sponsored organizations have reported increased losses on the physician enterprise over the last four years (Exhibit 5.1).

## Exhibit 5.1 Average Integrated Health System Loss per Physician

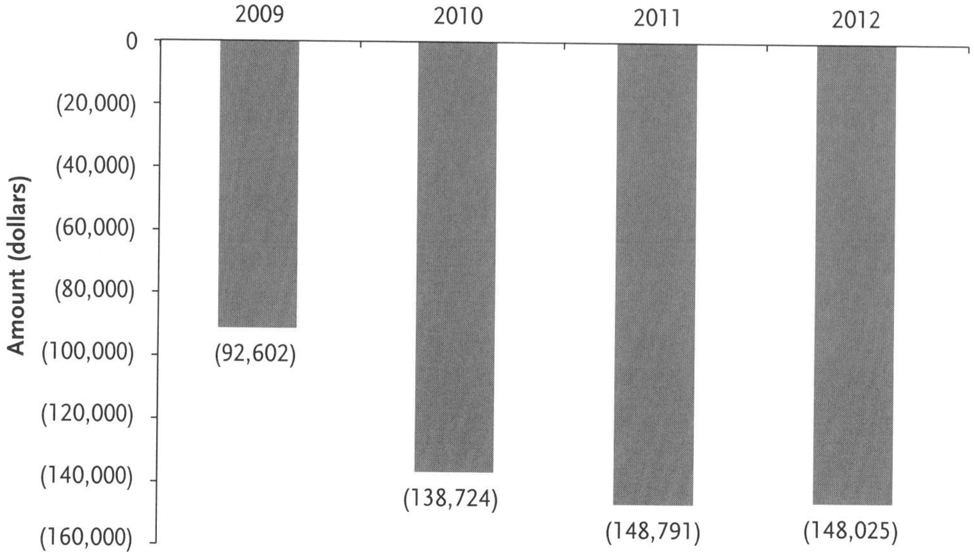

*Source*: Data from ECG Management Consultants, Inc. National Physician Compensation Surveys (www.ecgmc
.com/national-physician-compensation).

## BE CAREFUL WITH FINANCIAL ASSUMPTIONS

When a system encounters losses far exceeding the budget, the cause is seldom
isolated to operational failures. More often than not, the budget is built on faulty
assumptions that lead to unrealistic expectations, which in turn amplify the effect
of any implementation issues. Among the most common errors in assumption are
the following.

◆ **Dangerous assumption #1: Physician practices should remain at breakeven.** Big losses are difficult to understand if one assumes that because the
  physicians were breaking even prior to employment (collections – expenses =
  physician compensation), then the practice should be close to breakeven when
  owned by the hospital. In reality, costs go up and revenue goes down when
  a hospital affiliation is implemented. Cost increases associated with hospital
  employment include
  – system overhead allocations,
  – electronic health record (EHR) implementation,
  – physician compensation enhancements,
  – benefit increases,

- compliance requirements, and
- compensation for physician management and medical direction.

On the revenue side, hospital accounting practices often dictate that in-office ancillary services are credited to an ambulatory technical fee account rather than to physician revenue. Far from trivial, this amount can reduce what is reported as average physician revenue by 15 to 20 percent. The bottom-line impact of hospital employment can therefore be substantial even when physician work effort and visits remain unchanged.

- **Dangerous assumption #2: The hospital can manage physician practices more efficiently.** The thinking behind this assumption is that private practices and groups are poorly run and that any increased costs resulting from system affiliation should be more than balanced by gains in operating efficiency under hospital management. After all, the reasoning goes, the health system currently manages a large and diverse healthcare enterprise, so the physician business should be a simple add-on. This assumption is simply wrong. Independent physician practices may not have the latest and greatest management systems, and they may be unaware of (or ignore) some basic management principles, but they run as if every dollar spent comes out of the owners' pockets, which is in fact the case. Hospitals can often bring better management to medical groups, but they are rarely able to manage practices at lower cost.

- **Dangerous assumption #3: Physician practices will not change significantly.** Aided and abetted by assurances from hospital management, medical group physicians often expect that their practice will remain essentially unchanged after the acquisition. After all, it will have the same patients, the same office staff, the same locations, and so forth. They assume any changes will affect primarily the medical group board and administrative staff. However, if the new organization is going to be successful, it will involve fairly extensive changes in physician practices, including the introduction of patient care protocols, provider evaluations, documentation requirements, referral requirements, and training sessions, as well as changes in equipment, supplies, computer systems, and so on. Prior to executing the transaction, the physicians must understand what changes to their routines are likely and recognize that these changes are necessary for their long-term stability and success. The financial forecasts must reflect the reality that these changes can be stressful and may temporarily reduce productivity, especially with the implementation of a new EHR.

- **Dangerous assumption #4: New physicians will be busy quickly.** One of the advantages of an integrated system is having the capital to recruit and deploy new physicians quickly; this capital is a component of most physician-enterprise business plans. Particularly in the case of primary care, which has shortages in virtually all markets, financial forecasts commonly assume that a new practice will have a full panel of patients after six months, with a payer mix similar to that of other physicians in the enterprise. Except in special situations, 18 to 24 months is more realistic for a new practice to reach capacity, and the payer mix will be less favorable than what other employed primary care practices have. This slow start-up is common for many reasons, including community awareness, accessibility, acceptance within the community of other providers, and restrictions on certain payer types (e.g., Medicaid, Medicare). When new physician start-ups are planned, care should be taken to project a realistic ramp-up of visits and to hire new physicians at intervals to avoid inappropriate competition among providers within the same system (i.e., no more than one new physician in a specialty in any 18-month period).

These and other financial assumptions can mean that operating results will be significantly below budget regardless of the quality and efficiency of the group's management. Throughout the process, system leadership should question assumptions, understand the likely magnitude of capital requirements, and create reasonable expectations in the minds of all stakeholders, including administrators, physicians, and board members. For example, the board should understand that developing employed physician practices will require a significant amount of cash and that liquidity will likely suffer after the transaction is final. Establishing a communication plan, as discussed in Chapter 2, can be an effective tool to reduce misunderstanding and contentiousness related to the financial performance of the physician enterprise.

## RESPECTING THE CHALLENGES OF PHYSICIAN PRACTICE MANAGEMENT

Losses of the magnitude described above are seldom budgeted and are often vexing to system leadership and physicians alike. The reason is that hospitals and medical groups are fundamentally different businesses, with different goals and ways of operating. The following differences affect operational performance most directly:

◆ **Structure:** Hospital operations are highly centralized. Physician practices involve many small offices, frequently spread throughout the community.
◆ **Customer base:** Hospitals provide services to relatively few patients with clear needs for treatment. Physician offices see a large number of patients,

many of whom either are the "worried well" or have self-limiting illnesses or conditions.

◆ **Managers:** Hospitals have many professional administrators on staff. Most medical groups (other than the largest) have only support staff (accounting, billing), with management provided by the physicians, who determine everything from the length of their appointment slots to the brand of gauze that is used to treat wounds.

◆ **Size and scope:** Midsize hospitals have thousands of employees doing diverse tasks. Medical groups average fewer than four employees per physician in less varied roles.

◆ **Transactions:** Hospital bills typically average in the thousands of dollars. Physician office visits usually generate under $100.

◆ **Performance measures:** Key measures for physician performance are built around visits, relative value units (RVUs), and operating expenses per physician full-time equivalent (FTE). In the hospital, performance measures focus on admissions, diagnosis-related groups, and cost per adjusted bed day.

If hospital leaders understand from the outset that operating a medical group requires a different skill set than managing the hospital, many costly mistakes can be avoided. The attributes of an effective physician practice manager are discussed later in this chapter.

## MINIMIZING LOSSES

When faced with unacceptable losses in the physician enterprise, hospital leaders should explore three significant improvement opportunities:

1. Reduce operating costs
2. Adjust physician compensation
3. Enhance revenue

The biggest opportunities for margin improvement in physician practices are generally on the revenue side. Improvement in productivity and revenue cycle functions, including health plan contracting, often represents the greatest opportunity. In contrast, the largest opportunities in hospital performance improvement are mainly found in labor and nonlabor costs. The following discussion of each of these opportunities highlights those approaches that have the greatest potential impact on the bottom line.

## The Usual Suspect: Operating Costs

An obvious first step in dealing with unbudgeted losses is an in-depth review of operating costs. The following actions have the greatest potential for efficiency gains and cost savings for the system:

♦ Restructure clinical work flows
♦ Reconfigure space utilization to simplify patient and staff flows
♦ Optimize electronic tools, including health records
♦ Standardize order sets and other clinical practices
♦ Centralize supplies inventory and eliminate duplicate equipment
♦ Evaluate staffing models for best practices and sharing opportunities
♦ Capture economies of scale in IT infrastructure and services

The trick is not just in identifying what can be improved, but also in implementing and sustaining improvement initiatives. Managing physician practice expenses and overhead requires attention to detail as well as the standardization of processes across all practice sites. When physician practices move from independent to employed, the culture of expense management often fades away. Instead of a culture focused on "spending money as if it were your own," an attitude that treats expenses like "someone else's money" can emerge. Physicians anticipate little change to their practice, and hospitals frequently avoid standardizing processes for fear of alienating them.

Services that should be centralized across physician practices include IT system support and maintenance, revenue cycle activities, human resources (HR), physician compensation, and managed care contracting. Day-to-day operational activities are difficult to standardize in acquired practices because old habits are hard to break, and the physician or site coordinator can easily substitute work flows that they personally prefer. Functions affected can include appointment scheduling, registration, patient intake, coding and charge capture, patient discharge, referrals, prescription refills, and so forth. Challenging a practice's notion that "we are different" or "that really does not apply to us" or "our doctors prefer to do it a different way" is not easy. Physician practice managers may be able to persuade the practices to change voluntarily, but they must be prepared to insist on compliance when necessary.

The best time to implement new standardized processes is when a physician or group is considering becoming part of the employed physician enterprise. For existing practices, it may be necessary to retrofit operations, but the same concepts apply. Establishing appropriate expectations and a culture that cares about financial performance has three components:

1. **Operational review:** The purpose of the operational review is to understand and consider how the practice currently operates and the magnitude of the adjustments required to meet system standards. The review should include health plan contracts, revenue cycle, patient throughput and capacity, IT systems and infrastructure, staffing (levels, roles, competencies), and provider work standards.[1] A practice audit can be designed that includes work flow observations, a review of existing policies and procedures, an evaluation of existing management tools, and interviews of the providers and selected staff.

2. **Orientation of providers and staff:** Practice acquisition can be a worrisome proposition for both the physicians and the clinic staff, who may wonder if they have a future in the larger organization. Too often, efforts by physicians to protect their staff can create confusion and uncertainty. Staff are less willing to adopt and support standardized processes if they feel threatened and defensive. On-site meetings with practice staff can diffuse anxiety; management can answer their questions, engage them in the process, and support the cultural transition. Written materials, such as manuals and policy and procedure documents, should support and inform the on-site orientation rather than replace it. Physicians and staff should complete a structured orientation program before the implementation period to smooth the transition and initiate the relationship-building process.

3. **Assessment of practice manager and staff:** A sensitive yet important issue during the transition to system employment is the role of the physician's or group's office manager. On the negative side, this person may not have the skill set to function well under the new hierarchy, she may remain protective of "her" doctor, and she may be redundant because the system has other management talent. On the other hand, she may be an experienced and competent manager whose skills the system can use effectively. The value of having a strong practice manager in place throughout the integration process should not be underestimated. While the acquiring organization may be tempted to acquire the clinic first and review staffing competencies later, it should evaluate the legacy practice manager as early as possible in the process and not make any commitment to employ her before establishing that an appropriate role exists and that she has the skills necessary to transition the practice into the health system and assume that new role. Review of other staff members

is also important, to ensure that underperforming or disruptive staff members are not transitioned into the system's employment without exploring the options of reassignment or termination. If a program is already stuck with an underperforming practice manager or staff, aggressive action should be taken to either improve or replace these employees.

Although cost reduction frequently gets the lion's share of attention in a turnaround plan, cutting costs has only a limited role in fixing an ailing physician practice. The more significant opportunities are in rationalizing physician compensation and pursuing revenue enhancement initiatives.

## Bigger Returns, Tough Decisions: Rationalizing Physician Compensation

After an initial employment period, usually one or two years, the initial compensation plan is often reviewed and revised. Almost inevitably, deficits generated by relatively new employed groups are larger than budgeted, which drives the renegotiation of both the plan methodology and the amount of pay. In the early years of employing physicians, the hospital usually focuses on gathering up all interested physicians who meet very basic quality standards, and not on operating the group. When it comes time to renegotiate the initial contracts, financial viability is still an important driver, but organizational strategy also assumes a large role. This renegotiation is an opportunity not only to ensure that the compensation methodology (see Chapter 4 for details) is market based and sustainable but also to evaluate if the system has the right number of physicians in the right specialties, with the right quality standards and the right work ethic.

If the partnership between hospitals and physicians is going to be successful, hard decisions need to be made jointly by physician and hospital leaders. They must evaluate compensation levels, set and enforce performance expectations, and share a commitment to eliminating physicians who are marginal or underperforming. Examples of such difficult situations are presented in Exhibit 5.2.

The potential responses in these examples are not mutually exclusive, nor are they the only possible responses, but they demonstrate that meaningful solutions are likely to involve painful and unpopular actions. All too often, hospitals set general improvement goals with unspecified future sanctions and make only minor adjustments in near-term compensation. Contentiousness with the providers is avoided, but the operational structure and performance are unlikely to change. Meaningful and necessary reshaping of physician compensation remains among the

**Exhibit 5.2 Examples of Rationalizing Physician Compensation**

| Situation | Potential Responses |
|---|---|
| A PCP whose number of visits and RVUs have not exceeded the 35th percentile after two years of employment in the system has compensation guaranteed at the regional median. Community demand for primary care remains high. | ◆ Tie compensation to this provider's productivity (e.g., not to exceed the 35th percentile).<br>◆ Evaluate operational and other issues (e.g., access, location).<br>◆ Explore practice sharing with another provider. If the visit run rate is not at the median by the end of 18 months, terminate the employment arrangement. |
| A six-physician cardiology group was acquired one year ago, with substantial first-year compensation guarantees. The productivity of the group averages 40 percent of the regional median, while compensation is at the 70th percentile. | ◆ Reduce average compensation to reflect productivity within another 12 months.<br>◆ Develop a plan to improve productivity, or rightsize the group by consolidating volumes over fewer physicians. Expand marketing efforts for the cardiology service line, with employed physicians sharing financial risk. |

most difficult challenges facing integrated systems, but it is absolutely necessary for the success of the enterprise as a whole.

Restructuring compensation can only be done effectively if physician leadership is closely involved in the process. A compensation committee can be an especially effective structure for bringing together diverse perspectives and truly empowering physician leadership. Compensation committees have historically been convened on an ad hoc basis to recommend revisions to an existing compensation plan. This group deserves a much broader role, including understanding and managing the transition from production- to value-based provider compensation and providing guidance on the mix of physicians to be retained. The committee should be a standing one that includes physician leaders, hospital management, contracting staff, and practice administration, with broad authority to design, monitor, and revise physician compensation. The committee's charge should make it clear that compensation policies will reflect organizational strategy and follow compensation principles set by the governing body (see "Sample Compensation Principles" box).

## Sample Compensation Principles

- **Market competitive:** Funding must be adequate to attract and retain the best physicians.

- **Aligned incentives:** The highest degree of success is obtained when PCPs', specialists', and the hospital's incentives are mutually supportive.

- **Transitional:** An evolution to more sophisticated payment arrangements (e.g., shared savings, value based) should be promoted over time.

- **Sustainable:** Compensation should be aligned with overall financial performance.

- **Administratively feasible:** Metrics and incentives should be easily tracked and calculated.

- **Accountable:** Objective performance metrics agreed to in advance must drive variances in compensation.

- **Shared risk and reward:** The degree of reward available should correspond with the level of risk assumed.

Data transparency and effective communication are important operational keys to successfully engage physicians in compensation planning. Data transparency means more than that the source of data is known. It also means that performance improvement is explicitly expected; that physicians receive, review, and correctly interpret data on a regular basis; and that physicians are ranked by name according to performance. Effective communication includes providing a forum for feedback; connecting physician concerns to group action; informing physicians about new initiatives, quality and financial performance, and key decisions; and reinforcing the vision and strategy of the organization. Not coincidently, data transparency and effective communication are features that organizations need to develop if they are to become clinically integrated.

## Ongoing Opportunity: Revenue Enhancement

Given the current reimbursement environment, hospitals need to focus on physician productivity as well as on health plan payments to effectively manage revenue. Although less emphasis will be placed on productivity as reimbursement moves to more value-based arrangements, fee-for-service will still remain the dominant form of reimbursement for the next few years. Under the fee-for-service rubric, work

RVUs are the most common metric for evaluating physician productivity. Work RVUs provide a standard currency across physician practices and geographies, and they do a decent job of measuring work output within specialties.

For hospital-employed physician practices, coding and revenue cycle operations are basic functions that require careful management. Coding for physician services is often poorly understood by inpatient managers. The impact of coding on revenue is maximized in two ways: (1) by ensuring that the evaluation and management (E/M) code used is consistent with the documentation in the medical record and (2) by understanding how the coding frequency distribution compares to the market. An annual coding audit that includes a sample of each physician's charts protects the organization from a compliance perspective but can also uncover missed revenue opportunities. Larger groups (more than 50 physicians) should employ a certified coder or coders to provide ongoing feedback to physicians regarding coding and documentation opportunities. An individual physician's coding levels can be compared to those of other physicians in the same specialty using publicly available Medicare data or purchased surveys.

As an example, Exhibit 5.3 compares the coding practices of internist Dr. Gray for his established patients with the average of the internal medicine physicians within the enterprise. It reveals that, compared to other physicians in his specialty,

**Exhibit 5.3 Established Patient E/M Codes of Individual Physician Compared with Specialty Average**

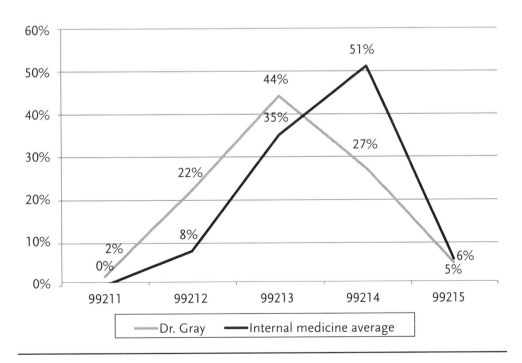

Dr. Gray undercodes established patient visits. Analysis shows that if Dr. Gray had the same coding distribution as the average, his gross revenue would increase by $68,000. Sharing this data with Dr. Gray and having a review process with a certified coder can increase his revenue to the appropriate level.

Physician revenue cycle management is another key competency required to run a successful physician practice. Too often, physician billing is managed through the hospital's receivables department. Major differences in coding, reimbursement policies, follow-up activity, and so on require specialized management practices. Best practices in physician revenue cycle are covered in Chapter 6.

Important opportunities may also be overlooked when negotiating with payers, because contracts for physician services can be a lower priority than contracts for hospital services. At a minimum, health systems need to develop a contracting strategy for physician services and make sure to take advantage of Medicare revenue opportunities (or to minimize penalties, as will soon be the case). Current Medicare incentive programs include the following:

- Physician Quality Reporting System (PQRS)
- Primary Care Incentive Payment (PCIP) Program (provides a 10 percent increase on the Medicare fee schedule for PCPs, in place from January 2011 through December 2015)
- EHR Incentive Program (meaningful use)
- Physician Value-Based Payment Modifier (proposed implementation in 2015 based on 2013 performance)

Chapter 11 discusses a detailed approach and best practices for physician commercial payer contracting.

More traditional business development initiatives should also not be overlooked. For example, provider work standards should be established to ensure that patient access is maintained. Work standards for a full-time physician commonly include the following:

- Minimum of 36 hours of patient contact per week
- At least 20 patients scheduled per 8-hour clinic day for PCPs

While the concept of work standards is straightforward—to establish norms of behavior for work hours and work effort—ensuring compliance with those standards depends on the culture of the physician group and the ability to put peer pressure on outliers.

In a similar vein, an important factor in building a medical practice is patient satisfaction. Despite the widespread use of satisfaction metrics for hospital patients, too few hospital-employed groups have adequate parameters for the patient experience or any routine measurement of patient satisfaction.

## TIPS AND TOOLS FOR OPERATIONAL IMPROVEMENT

Each physician group has unique characteristics and will, of course, have varying priorities for operational improvement initiatives. At the same time, certain operational elements apply to virtually all groups and can make the difference between success and failure. Specifically, the lack of attention to these elements makes meaningful operational improvement difficult or impossible. A short list of improvement priorities includes EHR, practice dashboards, group management, and physician leadership.

### EHR: Handle with Care

Vital, of course, is that all members of the physician group ultimately work from the same platform, and the process for reaching that goal cannot be an afterthought. A fully developed EHR and connected practice management (PM) system has three important functions: financial management, operations control, and medical and quality management. When implemented thoughtfully, an EHR is a powerful tool for improving efficiency, quality, and patient satisfaction. However, implementing an EHR in an integrated system is complex and expensive, and it is something that must be done well if the investment is to be justified. Integrated systems literally cannot afford to fail when implementing an EHR.

For this reason, detailed plans for the implementation should be developed when a hospital is in the early stages of physician enterprise development. In addition to the questions about system selection and design, policies should be established for how long the new physicians have to adopt the EHR and what adoption really means. Guidelines are needed regarding data conversion from the physician legacy system—will all data be converted, none, or some? Manually or electronically? By whom and for how much? Another important aspect of planning is the need to standardize processes and document who uses the EHR and for what purpose. Exhibit 5.4 presents a simplified sample matrix identifying the types of data that each individual may be responsible for capturing in the EHR/PM system in each major practice work flow category. In categories where more than one person has responsibility, the work flow needs to be defined (e.g., what parts of the exam is the RN going to perform rather than the physician, and under what circumstances?).

**Exhibit 5.4 Sample EHR/PM Responsibility Matrix**

| Work Flow Category | Patient Services Representative | Medical Assistant | Registered Nurse | Provider |
|---|:---:|:---:|:---:|:---:|
| Scheduling | X | X | | |
| Check-in | X | | | |
| Rooming | | X | X | |
| Provider exam | | | X | X |
| Procedures | | | | X |
| Orders | | | X | X |
| Referrals | X | X | X | X |
| Checkout | X | | | |
| Prescription refills | | X | X | |
| Telephone encounters | | | X | X |
| Results review | | | X | X |

EHR/PM systems are configured with a limited set of process options, and deviation from these options quickly results in ineffective practice operations that are time consuming and overly burdensome for the providers, the practice staff, and ultimately the patients. A table like the example in Exhibit 5.4 should be supplemented with details regarding when the information should be documented (e.g., prior to patient discharge, within 48 hours of the encounter), how it should be documented (e.g., template, free text, voice recognition, dictation), and potentially even where it should be documented (e.g., in the exam room, at the nursing station). The details of the system use policy should align with meaningful use requirements as well as with other quality or service initiatives that the organization is pursuing. Finally, as changes are made to processes during the evolution of the group, policies and procedures must be updated and training protocols must be revised. The key takeaway is that in starting up or optimizing an EHR, careful planning, standardization of processes, and maintenance of documentation are critically important to operate the group successfully.

Going beyond these basics, consideration should be given to likely future changes in ambulatory medicine and new IT requirements. Successful physician practices will provide opportunities for patients to participate in their own care. The group needs to support this evolution by making the appropriate technologies available, including

- electronic consults and e-mail messaging with providers;
- online appointment scheduling, registration, health risk assessments, visit summaries, and diagnostic testing results;
- online bill pay;
- point-of-service kiosk check-in and checkout;
- automated patient health outreach, including health maintenance reminders; and
- text message appointment reminders and notifications.

Much of this functionality is available in patient portals that are integrated with the health system's EHR/PM system. For the patient to interact effectively with not just one provider but his entire care team, clinical information spread across disparate systems should be made easily accessible by means of health information exchange or provider portal technologies. Finally, advanced tools within available systems should be implemented to support population health management and medical homes or coordinated care.

## Practice Dashboards: Turning Data into Information

Many hospital-employed physician groups have woefully inadequate capabilities for gathering and acting on management information regarding medical practice performance. Without such capabilities, improving operational performance is problematic at best. Creating a dashboard of operating statistics for each important stakeholder can be especially effective for focusing attention and facilitating needed change. Dashboards allow users to identify and evaluate organizational performance by measuring and reporting key metrics and indicators. An effective dashboard has the following characteristics:

- **Credibility**—The dashboard must be updated regularly and report accurately to be considered a viable decision support tool and to be used to effectively change behaviors.
- **Usability**—Structures must be in place to ensure the dashboard is continually populated and integrated into organizational strategy and management processes.
- **Actionability**—The metrics reported are specific and defined, such that the audience can take action to guide, stabilize, or improve performance.
- **Simplicity**—Dashboards can often become too complex and lead to information overload. The targeted audience should be able to quickly identify performance issues without wading through minutiae.

While all of these characteristics are important to incorporate in the development of any dashboard, other considerations are unique to the intended audience, which can include the board and system C-suite executives, the group administrator, site managers, specialty cohorts, or individual physicians. In each case, the key question is: What data are important for that particular person or group? The following are variables to include in designing dashboards for these stakeholders:

- **Type of report:** The type of report represented by a dashboard (e.g., strategic, operational) should mirror the type of responsibility of the intended audience within the organization.
- **Number of metrics:** The number of metrics should be limited to those performance indicators that are most relevant to the target audience.
- **Granularity of data:** Different audiences will require different levels of detail, based on their responsibilities for improvement.
- **Report frequency:** All audiences will require data on a regular basis to evaluate performance, but some data will not be needed or updated as frequently.

Exhibit 5.5 outlines common characteristics of dashboards designed for four unique audiences.

The metrics that are operationally relevant at each level will vary significantly. An individual physician needs to know how his performance compares to that of his colleagues each month, whereas the CEO needs to track performance by specialty cohort on a quarterly basis. Exhibit 5.6 presents the types of metrics that could be included in a clinic- or department-level dashboard. The selection of specific data elements is determined by the strategy and priorities of a given organization and

**Exhibit 5.5 Dashboard Characteristics**

| Audience | Type of Report | Number of Metrics | Granularity of Data | Report Frequency |
|----------|----------------|-------------------|---------------------|------------------|
| Board or CEO | Strategic | 1 to 5 | High-level summary | Quarterly |
| Vice president or senior director | Performance | 5 to 10 | Summary | Monthly |
| Site manager | Operational | 10 to 15 | Detailed | Daily or weekly |
| Physician | Performance or operational | 5 to 10 | Detailed | Monthly |

should reflect the numbers that are most directly related to physician performance, such as the number of patient visits, patient satisfaction, and quality of care.

Performance targets or benchmarks are the final piece of the dashboard, allowing users to quickly judge if performance is good or poor and improving or deteriorating. Targets are generally set in one of two ways: by comparing performance with internal goals or by identifying appropriate industry benchmarks. While industry benchmarks may provide a sense of an organization's strengths and weaknesses in relation to the marketplace and its competitors, they are limited in terms of comparability and reliability. Benchmarking to mediocrity, which results from using a regional or national average rather than a reasonable expectation for performance within a particular organization, should especially be avoided.

**Exhibit 5.6 Dashboard Metrics: Clinic or Department Level**

| Metric Category | Significance | Sample Measures |
|---|---|---|
| Productivity by physician | Identifies high and low performers | RVUs, net collections, visits |
| Compensation adjusted for productivity by physician | Serves as an indicator of the effectiveness of the compensation model and identifies high- and low-performing physicians | Compensation per work RVU |
| Panel size by physician (primary care only) | Provides an indicator of PCP productivity, supports business development and recruitment initiatives, and helps ensure appropriate levels of access to primary care for patients | Raw panel size, complexity-adjusted panel size |
| Staffing per physician FTE (clinic level) | Provides an indicator of costs and can be an effective overall gauge of a practice's or group's operational efficiency and financial health | Clinical staff per physician FTE, front-office staff per physician FTE |
| Patient satisfaction by physician | Shows management where opportunities exist to improve and share best practices in regard to patient satisfiers | Percentage of patients who would recommend this provider |
| Healthcare Effectiveness Data and Information Set (HEDIS) performance by PCP | Supports the identification of low and high performers to best inform incentive programs and disseminate best practices | Immunization status, screening rates, chronic condition management indicators |

*(continued)*

Exhibit 5.6 Dashboard Metrics: Clinic or Department Level *(Continued)*

| Metric Category | Significance | Sample Measures |
|---|---|---|
| Clinic access measures | Enable management to identify demand trends, operational inefficiencies, and potential recruitment needs | Day(s) out to the third next available appointment, referral access to specialists |
| Time available for scheduling per physician | Illustrates the level of activity and efficiency of the scheduling process within a practice and identifies an optimal supply of physicians in the practice and across the enterprise | Time available for scheduling per physician |
| Meaningful use objective thresholds by eligible professional | Indicate how close a physician is to achieving meaningful use goals (meaningful use dollars associated with the successful capture and reporting of these metrics are often budgeted to offset EHR costs) | Demographics recorded, smoking status indicated, vital signs reported |
| Customer service indicators | Serve as additional measurements of patient satisfaction and support the identification of process improvement opportunities | Patient visit throughput times, response times to patient messages and refill requests |

Exhibit 5.7 presents an example of a dashboard designed for a board or C-suite audience, highlighting a small number of aggregate-level metrics that can be used to monitor performance and support strategic decision making.

## Group Management: Special Skills Required

Managing a medical group is very different from managing a hospital or other healthcare facility. While the differences may be obvious, many hospitals persist in placing hospital managers in administrative roles within the medical group, most often resulting in greater operational losses and friction with the employed physicians. These issues are not related to a lack of intelligence or commitment but to the different skill set needed to effectively manage the physician enterprise.

Most hospital-employed physician enterprises incorporate two important management positions: the practice manager and the executive director. The physician

## Exhibit 5.7  Sample Dashboard for Board or C-Suite

| Current Year: Monthly FY 2013 | First Quarter | Second Quarter | Third Quarter | Fourth Quarter | Year-End Total |
|---|---|---|---|---|---|
| Gross Charges | $ 94,160,000 | $ 93,360,000 | $ 92,410,000 | $ 94,460,000 | $ 374,390,000 |
| **Payments** | | | | | |
| Medicare | $ 8,070,000 | $ 7,870,000 | $ 7,938,000 | $ 8,095,000 | $ 31,973,000 |
| Medicaid | 8,080,000 | 8,205,000 | 8,050,000 | 8,105,000 | 32,440,000 |
| Commercial | 19,465,000 | 18,560,000 | 18,835,000 | 19,240,000 | 76,100,000 |
| Self-Pay | 888,800 | 658,800 | 760,800 | 761,800 | 3,070,200 |
| Other | 871,320 | 1,021,320 | 912,220 | 1,364,084 | 4,168,944 |
| Total Payments | $ 37,375,120 | $ 36,315,120 | $ 36,496,020 | $ 37,565,884 | $ 147,752,144 |
| **Expenses** | | | | | |
| Nonphysician Compensation | $ 12,250,000 | $ 13,500,000 | $ 12,800,000 | $ 12,300,000 | $ 50,850,000 |
| Physician Compensation | 21,000,000 | 22,500,000 | 21,850,000 | 22,300,000 | 87,650,000 |
| Other Expenses | 12,970,000 | 11,860,000 | 12,360,000 | 10,320,000 | 47,510,000 |
| Total Expenses | 46,220,000 | 47,860,000 | 47,010,000 | 44,920,000 | 186,010,000 |
| Operating Income | $ (8,844,880) | $(11,544,880) | $(10,513,980) | $ (7,354,116) | $ (38,257,856) |
| Number of Physician FTEs | 215.5 | 217.5 | 238.8 | 236.5 | 236.5 |
| Loss Per Physician FTE | $ (41,044) | $ (53,080) | $ (44,028) | $ (31,096) | $ (161,767) |

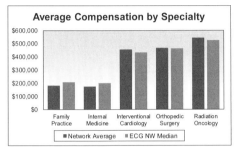

**Average Compensation by Specialty**

(Specialties: Family Practice, Internal Medicine, Interventional Cardiology, Orthopedic Surgery, Radiation Oncology — Network Average / ECG NW Median)

**Average Productivity by Specialty**

(Specialties: Family Practice, Internal Medicine, Interventional Cardiology, Orthopedic Surgery, Radiation Oncology — Network Average / ECG NW Median)

### Patient Satisfaction

| Survey Question | Average CAHPS Score | Peer Group Percentile Rank |
|---|---|---|
| Q1. Time physician spent with you. | 78.4 | 14 |
| Q2. Physician concern for your questions/worries. | 86.8 | 65 |
| Q3. Physician kept you informed. | 85 | 50 |
| Q4. Friendliness/courtesy of physician. | 86.7 | 18 |
| Q5. Skill of physician. | 94.5 | 89 |
| Q6. Physician treated you with respect. | 92.3 | 88 |
| Q7. Physician used language you understand. | 90.2 | 86 |

### HEDIS Measures

| Metric | Target | YTD Performance |
|---|---|---|
| Colorectal Cancer Screening | 65% | 72% |
| Breast Cancer Screening | 80% | 77% |
| Cervical Cancer Screening | 65% | 79% |
| Control of Hypertension | 75% | 83% |
| HbA1c Screening | 90% | 92% |
| HbA1c Control | 90% | 88% |
| LDL Screening | 80% | 85% |
| LDL Control | 80% | 81% |
| Cholesterol Management | 85% | 76% |
| Immunizations | 95% | 97% |

practice manager oversees the daily operations of one or more practices and is ultimately accountable for operational performance. Key responsibilities include

- training, supervision, and termination;
- front-end revenue cycle management, such as scheduling, registration, point-of-service cash collections, and coding and charge capture;
- analysis of practice activity and financial reports;
- quality program coordination and compliance;
- policy and procedure implementation and monitoring;
- facility management;
- supply and inventory management;
- patient care and customer service coordination; and
- practice site physician relations and satisfaction management.

These positions are most often filled by the most competent office managers from the acquired practices, with each manager responsible for a number of sites or specialties.

The second management position, the executive director of the employed practices, is often at a vice-president level in the system structure. The executive director is the person who oversees and directs all aspects of the physician enterprise, including

- centralized services, such as
  - HR,
  - receivables management,
  - purchasing,
  - payer contracting, and
  - legal services;
- budgeting and financial reporting;
- strategic planning and implementation;
- physician recruiting and on-boarding;
- policy and procedure development; and
- physician leadership development and liaison.

Two key aspects relating to this position deserve mention. First, many hospitals organize their centralized services (e.g., HR, purchasing) under the existing hospital department manager, with a dotted-line relationship to the executive director overseeing the physician practices. In essence, this structure sends a message that physician practices are a hospital service unit just like inpatient pediatrics or the operating room, and it fails to respect the different culture and business environment of the physician practices. Examples include an HR department that requires all staff to have hospital orientation (even employees who never set foot in the hospital) and other policies that create delays in bringing on new staff members, and a purchasing department that will not break cases or provide daily delivery, thus failing to accommodate the small inventories and multiple sites common to physician practices. These types of issues can be resolved over time, but if the system remains hospital-centric in the early years of the physician enterprise, significant operational difficulties are likely.

The second key aspect of the executive director position is the way its required skill set and priorities change over time. A clear progression of management needs is dictated by the maturity of the physician enterprise (Exhibit 5.8). For the majority of hospitals, the first priority is expansion (physician recruiting). The focus then moves to developing management competence (operations), followed by imple-

**Exhibit 5.8  Necessary Attributes for Physician Enterprise Leadership**

| | |
|---|---|
| Phase 1: Expansion | A sales-oriented manager who understands physician practices and has planning experience |
| Phase 2: Operational excellence | A financially oriented group practice manager with credibility among physicians |
| Phase 3: Clinical coordination | A physician who is experienced in quality metrics, is respected by physicians, and possesses effective social skills |
| Phase 4: Physician partnership | A system CEO and a physician partner who are committed to expanding physician roles in the organization and creating a collaborative culture |

menting clinical coordination, and, finally, incorporating physicians in all aspects of system operations and governance. Operational difficulties are likely to arise when the hospital does not recognize the changing demands of the enterprise or is unable to work through the layering of management skills.

Often, an administrator can be found who is capable of managing Phases 1 and 2 in Exhibit 5.8. The most frequent breakdowns occur when that person lacks experience in practice management. Phase 3 proves to be the most challenging because a physician is required, and she must develop effective working relationships with a wide range of providers. Many organizations get bogged down at this stage either because their vision of care coordination is limited or because they lack a suitable physician leader. Success during Phase 4 depends on the willingness of senior physician and administrative executives and the board to promote and financially support the changes needed to create a fully integrated healthcare enterprise. At this point, many integration initiatives encounter conflict between their strategic goals and the entrenched culture of the organization. Integration requires commitment and focus to work through these conflicts and form the new culture needed to sustain an integrated delivery system.

## Physician Leadership: It Takes a Team

Virtually all hospital integration initiatives include physicians in administrative capacities (e.g., medical director) and a physician advisory committee that ensures physicians are included in at least some of the decision-making processes. Necessary and important, these limited roles must evolve over time into a true partnership, with physicians being embedded in all operational, political, and clinical aspects of the integrated system. System development can stagnate if physicians are not both engaged and empowered in these three different spheres:

1. **Operational leadership:** When decisions about scheduling policies, equipment priorities, staffing needs, and so forth are made, the physician perspective needs to be made a priority. Physician leadership is especially important when establishing physician compensation and work standards and ensuring compliance with those standards. Most organizations have one or more physicians who are interested in practice management issues and are able to make a significant contribution to building the group.

2. **Political leadership:** Building consensus among physicians is a critical skill, and the political leader specializes in relationships and the shaping of opinion. Too often this skill is unrecognized, and only rarely does the physician leader in operational issues also understand the nuances of how to gain and keep physician support for needed initiatives. Physicians who have this perspective are recognized as opinion leaders and can be powerful in facilitating discussions and working through contentious issues between physicians and the system. They should be sought out and given a role in the governance structure of the enterprise or system.

3. **Clinical leadership:** As difficult as it may be, a transformation from traditional isolated care delivery models to coordinated care models is required if the hospital is to remain successful. This transformation cannot be carried out exclusively by healthcare administrators. The requisite skills focus on
   - determining and implementing new clinical standards,
   - improving IT systems to support population health management,
   - reconstructing operational processes to support coordination of patient care,
   - sharing data with peers to identify variation and opportunities for improvement, and
   - evaluating provider performance.

Leadership must come from physicians who are supported by clinical coordinators, with administrators and financial managers ensuring that clinical decisions are sustainable. A balance of administrative and medical perspectives is an important goal. A leadership team that includes physicians, nurses, and lay administrators can be structured in many ways, but a dyad management structure, which pairs a physician leader with a senior administrator, can be an effective option for managing clinical coordination (see Chapter 3 for additional information on dyad structures).

## THE BOTTOM LINE

Any system that wants to build an employed physician enterprise faces the very real challenge of broadening the organization's goals while ensuring that the practices are run as efficiently as possible. The experience of most systems is that the investment required is significantly higher than planned, imparting a sense of urgency and contentiousness to operational improvement initiatives. The key messages of this chapter are the following:

- Create appropriate expectations among key stakeholders from inception.
  - Hospital employment results in increased costs.
  - Physicians will have to adopt new behaviors as part of hospital affiliation.
  - Health system boards must understand the implications of physician employment.
- Make the tough choices that are necessary for success.
  - Hire experienced physician practice management professionals.
  - Be aggressive in standardizing procedures.
  - Target physician compensation to market levels, not above.
  - Set clear work expectations and productivity targets.
  - Terminate underperforming physicians.
- Empower and engage physicians in the design and operations of the enterprise.
  - Provide meaningful information and operational data at appropriate intervals.
  - Identify and nurture physician leaders, who may have strategic, political, or operational skills.
  - Listen carefully to physicians and practice management leaders.

## NOTE

1. Because of antitrust concerns, independent organizations must be careful not to directly share pricing information on health plan contracts.

# CHAPTER 6

# The Challenge of Professional Fee Billing

*Benjamin C. Colton, Curtis A. Mayse, and David A. Wofford*

HOSPITALS FREQUENTLY FIND that the urgency to complete a series of physician acquisitions can override the planning and infrastructure development needed to assimilate these practices effectively (see Chapter 1). As a result, many hospitals are left with a mixed bag of acquired practices that function much as they did prior to their acquisition. For managers who must oversee acquired practices, this scenario can become unmanageable quickly, and nowhere more clearly than in revenue cycle operations.

Historically, hospitals that have employed physician groups have tended to downplay the importance of professional fee billing—perhaps because inpatient and ancillary revenues were the dominant sources of income, and as long as the physicians were generating referrals and collecting most of their charges, all was well. However, as reimbursement tightens and a larger portion of revenue comes from ambulatory providers, every dollar counts—now more than ever. In addition to this financial consideration, the following have an impact on effective professional revenue cycle management:

◆ **Patient satisfaction:** Patients' billing experiences, whether with physicians or hospitals, affect the likelihood that they will return to that provider. However, patients typically have more opportunities to find alternative physicians than alternative hospitals. A mismanaged professional revenue cycle for acquired practices may lead to erroneous balances or statements, disparate standards and policies, and poor service—all fueling patient dissatisfaction and possibly attrition.

◆ **Provider compensation:** Providers both affect the revenue cycle process and are affected by it. Subpar controls and inconsistent policies can contribute to problems with charge capture and collections, which can in turn affect any provider compensation arrangements that are based on productivity. For this reason, revenue cycle performance can significantly damage hospital–provider relationships over time.

◆ **Regulatory compliance:** Since 2011, the Office of Inspector General (OIG) has included a focus on evaluation and management (E/M) services in its annual work plan. Compliance can create a great deal of risk for hospitals that have recently acquired physician practices, because (1) providers are frequently involved in coding their own services, and (2) many providers coming from private practice are not well versed regarding compliance considerations.

As the physician enterprise grows, so does the need to develop a level of infrastructure sophistication that is usually not found in smaller, independent practices. Unfortunately, the need for a well-functioning professional fee revenue cycle is not always recognized, one major reason being that the difficulty and complexity of getting it right is often underestimated. The common assumption is that billing is essentially the same for hospital and physician services and that expertise in one area automatically translates to effectiveness in the other. Although the professional fee and hospital revenue cycles have steps in common (e.g., collect patient data, document services rendered, generate a bill, follow up on unpaid accounts), hospital leaders are often surprised to discover that professional fee billing is in many ways just as complex as hospital billing and that it requires specialists with different skills and knowledge than for hospital billing. Industry benchmarks show that collecting professional fees costs two to five times as much as collecting hospital charges (i.e., approximately 4 to 10 percent of collections for physician fees versus 2 percent of collections for hospital services). This difference should not be surprising, considering the much larger charge basis for inpatient services, but it is often overlooked when calculating costs of physician services. Moreover, for physicians' practices, collections costs as a percentage of revenue can vary dramatically, depending on specialty, payer mix, and accounting practices. For example, primary care costs are often in the range of 8 to 10 percent of collections, while surgical specialties are commonly 5 to 6 percent. When preparing financial plans, organizations should be careful not to underestimate collections costs and should consider both specialty and payer mix when establishing performance benchmarks.

Additionally, the nature of physician practice operations presents reimbursement challenges that are not typically found in the hospital setting (Exhibit 6.1). The remainder of this chapter outlines the essential elements of a successful professional fee billing system.

**Exhibit 6.1  Features of Professional Fee Billing**

| Feature | Significance |
| --- | --- |
| High volume of claims (thousands per physician per year) | ◆ Sophisticated analytical capability is required to identify trends and troubleshoot issues. |
| Small claim size (a few hundred dollars on average) | ◆ Cost of billing, as a percentage of collections, is high.<br>◆ Anticipated payment can be less than the cost of collections efforts. |
| Provider involvement | ◆ Provider documentation directly determines billing levels and heavily influences reimbursement. |
| Collection of copayments at the time of service | ◆ Copayments constitute a significant portion of overall revenues.<br>◆ Collection is often assigned to staff who have other duties (e.g., patient scheduling, registration, check-in) and who may be reluctant to perform this function. |
| Decentralized operations | ◆ Significant effort is required to manage front-office functions effectively. |
| Different rules regarding coding, bundling, and so forth | ◆ Charge capture, error resolution, and insurance follow-up require highly specialized skills for each specialty. |

# OVERVIEW OF THE PROFESSIONAL FEE BILLING PROCESS

The revenue cycle is a complex process that couples with the clinical work flow to ensure that the practice is compensated for the services provided (Exhibit 6.2). Each step in this cycle builds on and informs the next and relies on the quality of data provided. Moreover, every step presents opportunities to improve performance, whether through lowering costs or increasing collections. A more detailed examination of this process (Exhibit 6.3) suggests major keys to success.

## Exhibit 6.2  Steps in the Revenue Cycle Process

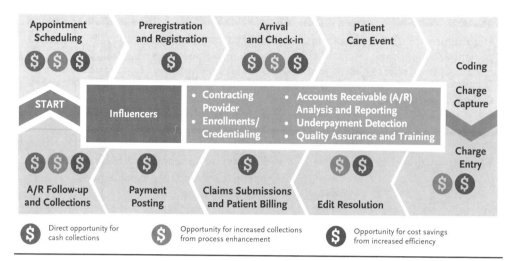

## Exhibit 6.3  Keys to a Successful Billing Cycle

| Step | Keys to Success |
|---|---|
| Appointment scheduling | ◆ Verifying or collecting registration data at time appointment is made<br>◆ Completing reminder calls<br>◆ Addressing past-due patient balances |
| Preregistration and registration | ◆ Verifying patient demographics and insurance coverage prior to visit<br>◆ Qualifying patients for financial aid prior to providing patient care, as necessary |
| Arrival and check-in | ◆ Validating patient information again<br>◆ Providing staff with training and tools necessary to collect patient balances at time of service |
| Coding and charge capture | ◆ Ensuring tools and processes are controlled and efficient<br>◆ Supporting staff and providers with ongoing coding and compliance education |
| Charge audit and manual entry | ◆ Establishing and adhering to coding and order entry procedure<br>◆ Actively pursuing missing charge reports |

*(continued)*

**Exhibit 6.3 Keys to a Successful Billing Cycle** *(Continued)*

| Step | Keys to Success |
|---|---|
| Edit resolution | ◆ Requiring edits to be resolved at point of origin<br>◆ Using robust technology to emulate payer's adjudication process prior to submission |
| Claims submissions and patient billing | ◆ Capitalizing on use of electronic claims submission<br>◆ Establishing controls to ensure timely submission |
| Payment posting | ◆ Using electronic remittances where possible<br>◆ Using lockbox service for sorting mail, depositing checks, and balancing cash and potentially for storing virtual records<br>◆ Training staff to recognize underpayments at time of posting<br>◆ Posting all remittances (including denials) to enable tracking of trends and issues<br>◆ Reconciling postings to deposits daily |
| A/R follow-up | ◆ Appropriately prioritizing follow-up activities<br>◆ Establishing consistent and effective follow-up procedures<br>◆ Developing working relationships with insurance representatives |
| Customer service and collections | ◆ Providing staff with tools and education necessary for success<br>◆ Establishing and consistently applying self-pay policies |

## HOW TO ORGANIZE IT

Regardless of the rationale for acquisition, the onus is on the acquiring organization to develop a consistent and coordinated billing model that can ensure efficient and effective revenue cycle management for employed physicians. While there is no magic formula, the most appropriate model should be easily scalable, improve primary revenue cycle performance, and support the organization's mission, vision, and strategic initiatives (e.g., rapid growth, high-quality patient service).

Prior to acquisition, practices are often accustomed to managing the full revenue cycle within the clinic, with clinic staff responsible for everything from eligibility verification to coding to patient collections. This model offers the significant advantage of giving clinic staff a sense of ownership, which is rooted in the recognition that the practice is a business and needs to be managed accordingly. However, on closer inspection, clinic-level billing operations are most often underperforming—coding is not compliant, accounts receivable (A/R) are not managed effectively, account follow-up is lacking, patient balances are left to age, and so on. This underperformance is typically the result of competing priorities: The pressure of responding to daily patient needs within the practice and the desire to get things done fast and cheap come into conflict with the need to carefully manage charges and collections. As a result, acquiring hospitals may find themselves wanting to improve the operation by consolidating some or all of the revenue cycle functions. Prior to making this decision, they must consider the benefits and consequences (Exhibit 6.4).

In the selection of a preferred billing model, the competencies of the acquiring hospital and the status of the acquired practice(s) are critical. If the acquisition is an early one and the hospital has never done professional fee billing for physicians, having the practice sites continue with their legacy billing systems under a single tax ID number may be appropriate. Decentralized billing may also be warranted when a new specialty is added to an existing group. For example, if an orthopedic group with a sophisticated billing system and experienced staff is acquired, adding this practice to a centralized primary care billing operation may not make sense, at least in the near term.

Decentralized models may be appropriate in the early stage of enterprise development, but as the organization grows, so does the need for a centralized and functionally organized billing office to ensure each task is addressed and economies of scale are achieved (i.e., costs are reduced). Ideally, practice sites should focus on creating a positive experience for patients and perform only those revenue cycle tasks that cannot be centralized (e.g., copayment collection). A centralized approach can increase expertise, reduce errors, provide flexibility for new payment methodologies, and minimize exposure to compliance issues.

Most organizations find success in deploying a hybrid strategy that leverages economies of scale while simultaneously locating functional responsibilities where they can be serviced most efficiently (see Exhibit 6.5 for an example). The rationale for a hybrid model is that better revenue cycle performance typically results when all billing functions follow common guiding principles—most easily accomplished when these functions, and the staff who perform them, are managed as part of a single team. In a hybrid model (e.g., Exhibit 6.5), functions that do not require face-to-face patient or physician interaction are centralized; however, locally managed clinical support staff are still expected to adhere to common revenue cycle policy. This reporting relationship ensures that financial matters do not become a secondary priority, particularly among staff who also have patient-facing duties, such as check-in.

Controls, performance standards, and work standards should be established to ensure that protocols are followed at all sites. The clinic should be held responsible for certain tasks (Exhibit 6.6). Moreover, when possible, edits and denials related to front-office errors should be routed back to the clinic for resolution. While this process may increase the lag time for correction, it ensures that the clinic staff know

**Exhibit 6.4  Comparison of Billing Models**

| Billing Model | Description | Advantages | Disadvantages |
|---|---|---|---|
| Centralized | Majority of billing functions are completed in a central business office (CBO) | ◆ Economies of scale<br>◆ Consistency<br>◆ Dedicated expertise<br>◆ Standardized reporting and monitoring<br>◆ Opportunities for enhanced IT systems and resources | ◆ Increased physician billing and response lag times<br>◆ Potential for higher billing costs, driven by investments in technology and additional functions (e.g., low-payment detection)<br>◆ Potential for "not my job" mind-set from front-office staff<br>◆ Greatest potential for clinic dissatisfaction if cash collections deteriorate |
| Hybrid | Some functions (e.g., coding, charge capture or entry, copayment posting) are completed at the site of service, while remaining functions are completed at the CBO | ◆ Clinic ownership of the revenue-generation process<br>◆ Prompt resolution of physician-driven errors<br>◆ Expertise and economies of scale in back-office operations | ◆ Additional training, reporting, and control tools required<br>◆ Potential staffing inefficiencies<br>◆ Detailed planning required for deployment of coding and charge entry staff |
| Decentralized | Majority of billing functions are completed or managed at the site of service (i.e., each practice maintains a small business office) | ◆ Site-level control<br>◆ Close relationship with patients and physicians, creating ownership<br>◆ Prompt resolution of physician-driven errors | ◆ Disparate standards and processes<br>◆ Staffing inefficiencies<br>◆ Billing management expertise required in each decentralized unit<br>◆ Not easily scalable |
| Outsourced | Functional areas (typically back-office functions) are managed by a third party | ◆ Organization free to focus on core competencies (e.g., patient service) | ◆ Third parties less apt to "care" as much about patients<br>◆ Premium on billing services |

## Exhibit 6.5  Suggested Delineation of Revenue Cycle Responsibilities

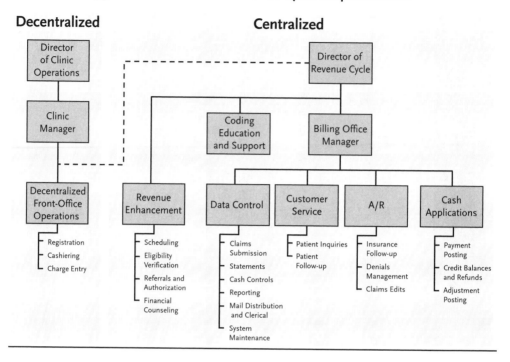

## Exhibit 6.6  Revenue Cycle Activities and Controls in the Clinic

| Function | Control |
|---|---|
| Registration and demographics verification | ◆ Last verification date<br>◆ Registration edits or denials rate |
| Eligibility verification* | ◆ Eligibility denials rate |
| Authorization verification* | ◆ Referral authorization denials rate |
| Time-of-service collections | ◆ Copayment collections rate<br>◆ Time-of-service payments as a percentage of total cash |
| Charity care and cash discounts | ◆ Audit process |
| Coding, charge capture, and charge submission | ◆ Charge lag |

*Some organizations find efficiency in centrally managing eligibility verification and the referral authorization process. Nevertheless, even with a centralized team, the front desk is the last safety net to confirm whether a patient is eligible to see the provider and should confirm that the centralized activities have been completed.

about their errors and resolve them, helping them to reduce future errors and avoid sloppy work based on the belief that someone will fix it on the back end.

On the back end of the revenue cycle, hospital-based organizations are often tempted to merge facility and professional fee billing operations. This is generally not a good idea. While the two operations have some similarities, they are sufficiently different that they require specialization, and skill in hospital billing is no guarantee of success at physician billing. More important, hospital billing tends to deal with lower volumes of high-dollar claims, whereas professional fee billing deals with large volumes of smaller-value claims. If the two operations are intermingled, hospital billing will almost certainly take priority at the expense of professional fee billing.

To ensure consistency (e.g., policy adherence) across the health system, some organizations create a position for a revenue cycle executive who is responsible for billing operations across the whole enterprise. Still, in addition to maintaining separate billing teams, appropriate and distinct goals should be established for hospital and professional fee operations.

## MAKE OR BUY

System-owned physician groups sometimes outsource most revenue cycle operations to vendors as a means of accessing advanced practice management capabilities more quickly or more economically than they could if they developed them on their own. Outsourcing can be particularly advantageous when the group is anticipating rapid growth and the need for scalability is great. Another advantage is that billing services frequently offer specialty-specific expertise in billing and coding, which can be valuable in specialties with unique requirements, such as anesthesiology and radiology. Outsourcing also decreases the number of internal staff, reducing human resources issues and the administrative burden on the system. For all these reasons, outsourcing can be an attractive option for organizations that lack the infrastructure or management expertise needed to run a large, consolidated billing shop and do not wish to devote the energy and resources to develop one in-house.

Three factors must be considered when deciding whether outsourcing of the revenue cycle is appropriate: (1) the current staff's competence in professional fee billing, (2) the adequacy of the current electronic health record (EHR) or billing system, and (3) the ability of the current staff and systems to expand with the growth of the physician enterprise. If two or more of these areas have significant weaknesses that cannot be repaired quickly, then outsourcing the revenue cycle function is likely the best option. Many health systems will also consider outsourcing if the current in-house costs are higher than benchmarks or if collections percentages have deteriorated.

However, outsourced billing is by no means a panacea, and the buyer should proceed with caution when selecting a billing agency. One of the most common misperceptions about outsourcing the billing operation is that it provides a turnkey solution requiring little involvement from the clinic or system staff. Although less hands-on involvement is needed when the billing operation is outsourced (e.g., for staff recruiting and training), the requirement does not go away altogether, and the relationship with the billing agency demands ongoing attention. Most billing agencies are paid a percentage of collections, which would appear to align incentives but may not always work in practice. Because the billing company gets to keep only a small fraction of what it collects, claims that are difficult to collect are time-consuming money losers. The company has an incentive to write them off rather than invest great effort for a small and uncertain return.

Clearly, specific policies and procedures need to be negotiated as part of the contract with a billing agency to avoid any conflicts. Exhibit 6.7 provides a checklist of key considerations when organizing an outsourcing partnership.

Before executing a contract, health systems should of course talk with the billing agency's existing customers about their experience with the agency and listen carefully to ascertain the extent of the users' familiarity with the agency's performance. Many happy customers simply don't know what kind of job their billing agency is doing. An additional consideration is how information will be kept secure from competitors and potential competitors. What procedures are in place to ensure that the billing agency will never disclose the practice's service volumes, progress, and

### Exhibit 6.7 Checklist for Outsourcing Revenue Cycle Functions

| | |
|---|---|
| Defined policies, procedures, work standards, and business rules | ✓ |
| Measurable milestones and deliverables | ✓ |
| Regular reporting and oversight to ensure adherence to the agreement | ✓ |
| Clear understanding of the outsourcing team's size, skill set, commitment, and competing responsibilities | ✓ |
| Seamlessness for patients (i.e., the billing service should seem like an extension of the practice) | ✓ |
| Near-seamless integration with the clinical enterprise (i.e., handoffs with the billing service, both physical and electronic, should be controlled and efficient) | ✓ |
| Term of the agreement and termination provisions | ✓ |
| Dispute resolution procedures | ✓ |

plans for expansion to third parties? Finally, organizations need to keep in mind that a billing agency's ultimate incentive to perform is the fact that customers can take their business elsewhere if things don't work out. Sound exit provisions (e.g., ownership of the data, contract termination upon minimum net collections rate or maximum days in A/R) will ensure that the agreement can be smoothly terminated if necessary.

Contracting with a billing agency does not have to be an all-or-nothing decision—portions of the revenue cycle can be outsourced. While the best practice is still to manage the patient portion internally, outsourcing selected functions (e.g., customer service, patient balance follow-up) or those that require specialized expertise (e.g., coding) can be beneficial under the right conditions.

## ORGANIZATION OF AN APPROPRIATE CODING AND COMPLIANCE MODEL

The coding process is no easy task—more than 7,500 CPT codes and 17,000 ICD-9 diagnosis codes are currently available, and a myriad of complex payer and regulatory guidelines must be followed. Moreover, physician practices use a wide array of resources and processes to complete this work; some groups require physicians to select codes via an EHR or encounter form, while others use support staff to abstract directly from the medical record. Each approach has its benefits and limitations. Although the challenges are not new—inadequate attention to coding has always had the potential for high-cost repercussions (e.g., increased billing lag, unnecessary denials)—the OIG's recent focus on E/M coding signals the likelihood of increased scrutiny of physician billing in the ambulatory setting, adding the high costs for audits and recoupment to the list.

Unfortunately, developing an appropriately sized and equipped coding support structure can be tricky for many hospital-based physician groups. The tug-of-war that occurs as a result of trying to maximize revenue without crossing any compliance boundaries can be daunting, especially when physician compensation is based on productivity—some providers and management may even view the implementation of a coding oversight function as antagonistic. As the risk of being charged with overcoding is coupled with revenue loss due to undercoding, many organizations are now examining the adequacy of their coding infrastructure.

Experience shows that better-performing organizations maintain coding programs that are designed to balance regulatory compliance with revenue maximization and take several key attributes into consideration (Exhibit 6.8). In short, they make sure the documentation for each visit supports the coding submitted for payment.

**Exhibit 6.8  Coding and Compliance Considerations**

| Attribute | Consideration |
|---|---|
| Consistent coding and compliance policies tailored to the practice | ◆ Coding and compliance policies should be established based on payer- or specialty-specific guidelines. Some payers reimburse for certain coding events that Medicare does not—organizations should not forfeit this opportunity because of an unnecessarily rigid compliance program.<br>◆ A communication plan should be developed to articulate the source/rationale for these policies and keep providers informed, ensuring their buy-in and support. |
| Proactive and reactive provider education | ◆ A consistent, documented communication loop should be established between providers and coders, including real-time feedback on their error trends, how to improve, and any changes to their charges.<br>◆ Providers should receive coding education, both regular (e.g., semiannual classes) and ongoing (e.g., tips and tricks), to better understand compliance expectations and opportunities to improve documentation for optimal reimbursement. |
| Regular compliance audits | ◆ Periodic audits should be completed for each provider (or abstracting coder).<br>◆ Providers performing below a predefined accuracy rate (e.g., 75 to 80 percent) should be coached and re-audited within a probationary period.<br>◆ Audits should be rooted in compliance, not revenue maximization. |
| Qualified support staff | ◆ Certified coders should be employed, where possible, to assist with abstraction, review, education, and audit. Because certification does not mean expertise, coders need to be appropriately evaluated and should demonstrate experience in their assigned specialty.<br>◆ Annual education should be provided for each team member.<br>◆ Not all coders are created equal. Some are exceptionally skilled at abstracting chart notes into CPT and ICD-9 coding but lack appropriate communication skills, while others are more equipped to train and educate.<br>◆ In the event that certified coders or specialty-specific experts are not available, outsourcing should be considered. |

Developing a function-based model, where coders are deployed based on their skill sets and expertise to ensure the right people are doing the right work, will ensure optimal coding performance. In this model, the production team and audit team provide trends and feedback to members of the education team, who in turn are responsible for communicating with the providers (Exhibit 6.9). Given that each team is responsible for defined tasks in the coding process, this model enables consistency, quality, and the ability to measure and monitor results. Work standards and performance expectations should be established to confirm adherence to policies and protocols and to ensure proper management of work volumes and backlogs.

The audit team reports to a separate authority from the rest of the coders to ensure that charts are reviewed from a purely compliance-focused perspective, not from the standpoint of the revenue opportunity. Despite the segregation of duties, however, all members of the infrastructure must work from a common set of policies, and the teams should be led by qualified individuals with deep coding expertise.

Appropriate investment in coding and compliance (whether internally developed or outsourced) will ensure that the charge submission process is efficient, claims are billed and adjudicated appropriately, and risk and subsequent expense are mitigated. These enhancements will also result in patient and provider satisfaction.

## A WORD ON TECHNOLOGY

Chapters 5 and 9 discuss issues and opportunities in technology and physician employment. The impact that related decisions can have on the revenue cycle is also important. While leaving acquired practices on their existing systems may be appropriate in the short term, doing so can quickly go awry. Maintaining disparate systems challenges scale economies, the ability to monitor performance across multiple practices, and the prompt identification of problems in the revenue cycle. The most effective organizations transition all acquired practices to a single, robust practice management system that

- regulates a consistent approach to primary work flows (e.g., registration and demographics collection, eligibility verification, A/R follow-up);
- provides automation to facilitate the billing flow (e.g., electronic remittance posting, prioritized work queues);
- enables the management of all work flows at the site of service and remotely (e.g., centralized business office, scheduling call center);

**Exhibit 6.9 Sample Coding Model**

## Best-Practice Coding Model

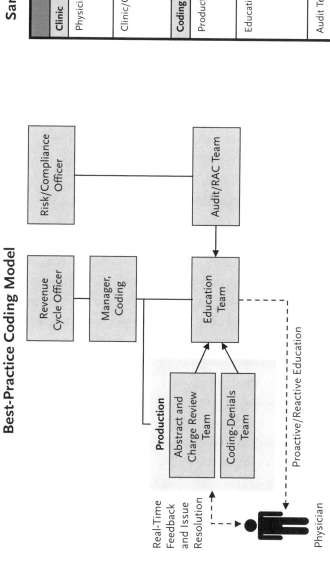

## Sample Roles and Responsibilities

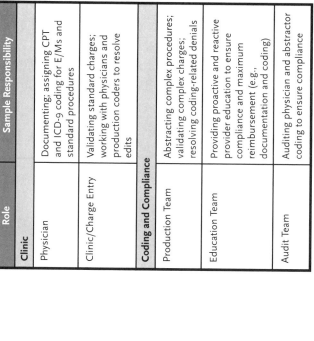

| Role | Sample Responsibility |
|---|---|
| **Clinic** | |
| Physician | Documenting; assigning CPT and ICD-9 coding for E/Ms and standard procedures |
| Clinic/Charge Entry | Validating standard charges; working with physicians and production coders to resolve edits |
| **Coding and Compliance** | |
| Production Team | Abstracting complex procedures; validating complex charges; resolving coding-related denials |
| Education Team | Providing proactive and reactive provider education to ensure compliance and maximum reimbursement (e.g., documentation and coding) |
| Audit Team | Auditing physician and abstractor coding to ensure compliance |

- allows for easy segmentation of performance where multiple tax IDs are in use (e.g., charge and collections volumes, A/R), while still creating efficient work queues that enable staff to manage billing effectively;
- allows for submission and management of both CMS-1500 and UB-04 claim forms to accommodate provider-based billing;
- offers the ability to monitor whether payments are in accordance with contract terms; and
- integrates with an EHR.

Moreover, maintaining a single system will enable the organization to efficiently navigate (or at least prepare for) the changing regulatory environment (e.g., HITECH/ARRA, ICD-10, payment reform). Implementing necessary regulatory changes across multiple platforms has the potential for being unmanageable.


## MINDING THE STORE

### It's a Numbers Game

Given the complexity of professional fee billing, many potential failure points can have an adverse impact on cash flow and may go unnoticed if the process is not monitored carefully. Fortunately, the nature of the professional fee revenue cycle is conducive to effective oversight, because it involves a high volume of claims that are processed through a sequence of discrete steps that are readily quantified and analyzed. As a result, troubleshooting problems can be very manageable, provided that the necessary analytical infrastructure is in place. This infrastructure needs to provide the following elements:

- The ability to actively track financial (e.g., charges, collections, aged A/R), performance (e.g., collections rates, denials trending), and productivity (i.e., staff and provider) metrics to manage the physician enterprise
- A hierarchical management reporting suite that can be reviewed at the provider, practice, and system levels (a daily, weekly, or monthly dashboard should be made available to all relevant stakeholders; see Chapter 5 for a discussion of the dashboard's content)
- A reporting package that includes relevant goals and benchmarks in dashboard reports to monitor performance
- End users or billing staff who have the analytical skills needed to interpret and apply the data

Relentless attention to detail and persistence in following established protocols are keys to success. As the physician enterprise grows in size and complexity, the ability to manage the revenue cycle "by the numbers" becomes ever more important. However, surprisingly few physician organizations have the degree of infrastructure sophistication needed to perform this function effectively. While recent vendor advances have resulted in more robust "canned" reporting, most organizations still rely heavily on analysts to populate dashboards, if reporting is done at all.

## What to Look For

Most organizations are well acquainted with basic revenue cycle performance metrics, such as days in A/R, aged A/R, and gross and net collections rates. These metrics provide a very quick assessment of the overall effectiveness of the revenue cycle and can indicate where a problem exists. However, the usefulness of these measures is limited because they are not actionable; that is, they reveal the outcome of the revenue cycle process but do not entail direct management of the process itself. By the time an issue shows up in these metrics, the problem has existed for some time and is likely to be bigger than it initially appears. Therefore, monitoring each phase of the process is necessary so that issues can be identified and corrected early on.

The following are some of the key metrics that are often overlooked but are essential to ensuring a smoothly functioning revenue cycle:

### Days Lag in Posting and Unposted Charges
These two closely related metrics measure the effectiveness of entering charges into the billing system. *Days lag in posting* can be measured only after charges have actually been posted. *Unposted charges* are measured by the number of patient encounters that have occurred (reported as "arrived") but for which no charge has been posted. An issue common to both metrics is that physicians often do not complete their documentation in a timely manner, thereby preventing charges from posting. Such delays are surprisingly pervasive and persistent, with some physicians routinely taking weeks to close their encounters. In an electronic environment, a variety of factors may hinder the data flow from the EHR to the billing system and cause further delays. The equivalent issue in a paper-based environment would be delays in submitting fee tickets for manual posting or backlogs in manually entering charges.

These metrics are important because delays in posting charges not only affect the timing of cash receipts but can also, in extreme cases, prevent payment altogether if timely filing requirements are not met. In manual posting, these delays often signal a lack of accountability for fee tickets. Furthermore, if the delays are caused by physicians not documenting care in a timely fashion, the quality of care can be affected. As a general guideline, organizations with EHRs should expect charges to post within 24 hours, and those working in a paper-based environment should expect posting within 72 hours.

### Claims in Edit

Most professional fee billing information systems have native functionality that scrubs claims to identify billing errors, so that the errors can be corrected before the claims are submitted to payers. Errors detected before each claim leaves the organization can be corrected more quickly, and cash flow will be enhanced. The practice management information system typically reviews these claims according to rules that the organization defines, assigning codes to identify the nature of the error (e.g., coding, registration, lack of a referral authorization). Monitoring the volume of claims that are held in edit is essential to identify recurring work flow issues that lead to claims errors, to manage backlogs in the resolution process, and to prevent interruptions in cash flow. To monitor the claims effectively, the claims edits must be assigned codes that can be readily translated into real-world terms so that end users understand what the code means and what corrective action needs to be taken (e.g., demographic errors may require that front-end staff be trained in the use of special characters in the address field). Additionally, these edits must reflect the rules that payers use in adjudicating claims. Keeping the edits up-to-date requires constant monitoring so that stale edits are removed and new edits are created as needed.

In addition to monitoring the number of claims in edit at any given time, expressing this number relative to some indicator of volume (e.g., as a percentage of weekly or daily claims) is helpful. Industry benchmarks are not typically used for this function, because they exist for internal use only and because organizations use claims edits to different extents. For example, some clinics hold all claims in edit as part of the normal work flow.

### Rejected and Denied Claims

Just as the internal edit process intercepts claims errors according to rules defined by the organization, payers (and claims clearinghouses) apply rules-based logic in adjudicating claims and reject or deny claims under certain conditions. The difference between rejected and denied claims is largely semantic; however, most organizations use *rejections* to describe claims that have been returned as incomplete or in need of correction and *denials* for claims that have been determined to be not reimbursable, even though they are often appealed and paid.

Because rejections and denials result in reimbursement delays, the volume of claims in each category at any given time is obviously an important metric to monitor and manage. Additionally, the rates of rejection and denial are important indicators of recurring issues related to registration, coding, referral authorization, and other functions within the revenue cycle. Ideally, the rates are based on the percentage of claims that are rejected or denied the first time they are submitted. Better-performing organizations are able to maintain a first-time rejection rate below 5 percent (or alternatively, a clean claims rate greater than 95 percent). To reduce this rate, issues should be tracked to their root cause and addressed before the error is made.

### Administrative Adjustments (Write-Offs)

Like facility fees, professional fees are occasionally written off when claims are determined to be not reimbursable, when collections efforts have been exhausted, or when patients have complaints about their bills. The temptation to write off charges can be strong, either because the write-off makes the A/R balance look better or because it is an easy way to placate a dissatisfied patient. Accordingly, management controls need to be put in place to prevent inappropriate write-offs as well as to monitor the volume of write-offs that are occurring. Monitoring write-offs requires the ability to distinguish between administrative adjustments and the much larger volume of contractual adjustments (billed charges less contracted payment) that are applied by payers. Although most practice management systems have this capability, it is often not used, resulting in aggregate reporting without administrative adjustments being isolated and monitored.

### Staff Productivity

Like monitoring throughput and error rates at each stage of the revenue cycle process, tracking the productivity of individual employees is important. The metric applied will vary based on the employee's role, but most functions involve discrete units that can be measured readily. Examples include the number of

- patients registered per day,
- patients checked in,
- insurance authorizations obtained,
- encounters coded,
- edits or rejections resolved, and
- payments posted.

The size of backlog, or work queue, for each function also needs to be monitored to ensure effective throughput.

Despite the importance of measuring and monitoring billing staff productivity, most organizations do not effectively track staff performance because of the effort required or the lack of applicable productivity benchmarks. Although external benchmarks are difficult to come by, internal benchmarks can be derived from the productivity of better-performing employees. Also, while this type of monitoring requires effort, it is the only way to determine appropriate staffing levels and to evaluate the performance of team members. In the absence of monitoring, staffing decisions are based on a general, subjective sense of how busy people seem to be, which is a recipe for inefficiency.

## STAKEHOLDER ENGAGEMENT

Because the billing office does not operate in isolation, other stakeholders must be involved in the management of the revenue cycle function. What happens in the clinics during scheduling, registration, insurance verification, and coding and charge capture has a dramatic impact on how quickly, how much, and even whether reimbursement is received for a clinical service. Therefore, clinic staff, physicians, and operations and medical leadership need effective information on the performance of the revenue cycle and their roles within it. This information is typically provided in two ways: management reviews and provider education.

### Management Reviews

During management reviews, the clinic managers and their operations leadership review the revenue cycle metrics, paying particular attention to the areas they influence, including

* collection of copayments and outstanding balances at the front desk,
* claims edits and rejections relating to registration errors, and
* delays in charge posting and unposted charges.

No single correct approach exists for conducting these reviews. In general, however, management reviews should take place fairly frequently, perhaps monthly, to address systemic issues as they arise. These meetings are best held in person and are greatly facilitated by the use of graphics (as opposed to page after page of tabular data). For the meetings to be effective, they must be attended by operations leadership, and these leaders must be invested in establishing accountability for the revenue cycle functions within their purview.

### Provider Education

The primary purpose of provider education is to help providers code services in a way that will minimize rejections, maximize legitimate charge capture, and avoid compliance complications. Because physicians' schedules do not allow a lot of time for meetings, education sessions are generally conducted less frequently than management reviews, perhaps semiannually. For the meetings to be effective, they must supply information that is relevant to the individual physician, ideally physician-level data about rejections, charge capture opportunities, and compliance issues.

## THE BOTTOM LINE

The challenges of developing an effective professional fee revenue cycle process—and the consequences of not getting it right—are often not adequately appreciated by hospitals that acquire physician practices. This is understandable, because the revenue cycle is more complicated and difficult than is usually assumed and something most managers want to avoid. It is hard to get past the belief that professional fee billing is boring work, but the reality is that it requires sophisticated leadership skills, including strategic vision, organizational design, management discipline, and infrastructure development. Most important, the impact of a well-run system on the bottom line of the organization can be enormous. Developing a smoothly functioning process is well worth the time and attention it requires.

Part II


# ALTERNATIVE ALIGNMENT MODELS

# CHAPTER 7

# Joint Ventures and Clinical Comanagement Arrangements

*John N. Fink*

HOSPITAL EMPLOYMENT OF physicians potentially represents the ultimate form of integration because it creates a single economic entity that can offer unified payer contracting, facilitate care management, pursue cost containment, and promote the integrated organization's long-term competitiveness. These attributes, combined with an uncertain economic climate for physicians, have caused rapid growth in both the number of hospitals that employ physicians and the number of employed physicians. However, other types of integration initiatives can be effective in achieving the same goals. Two of these alternatives are joint ventures (JVs) and clinical comanagement arrangements. JVs generally improve alignment on the ambulatory side, while comanagement arrangements improve alignment for inpatient and outpatient services. By using either or both alignment models, community hospitals are able to achieve many of the benefits associated with physician employment. This chapter summarizes key elements of JVs and comanagement arrangements, success factors in establishing and maintaining these arrangements, and ways they can be used together to improve alignment for a service line.

## THE BASICS

With the flurry of activity that surrounds physician employment, hospitals sometimes forget that not all physicians need or want to be employed and that most hospitals cannot prosper if employment is their only approach to aligning with physicians. On the physician side, reasons to remain outside of hospital employment include the following:

- Risk of losing patients or referrals
- Loss of autonomy and control over the practice
- Concern about the long-term viability of the new relationship
- Lack of consensus among medical group partners
- Absence of trust in hospital leadership

From the hospital's perspective, physician employment may not be an ideal strategy for many reasons, including the following:

- A single hospital market, with a stable physician supply
- Little or no interest from physicians
- Lack of capital to create and sustain a physician employment initiative
- Intractable opposition from board or medical staff
- Legal or regulatory restrictions
- Fierce recruitment competition

Whether they decide to pursue an employment option or not, hospitals must realize that having meaningful alignment options for members of their medical staff is critical to their long-term success. Specifically, success under value-based arrangements will hinge on the ability to work collaboratively with physicians on improving the quality and affordability of care.

Therefore, both physicians who choose not to be employed and hospitals in most communities are interested in developing nonemployment options to respond to the changes that a growing consensus agrees are coming. JVs and comanagement opportunities may be valuable vehicles for developing the necessary partnerships between hospitals and physicians.

The "integration lite" strategies of the past, such as medical directorships, quality committees, and joint task forces, are clearly not adequate to meet the requirements of payment reform. Effective integration strategies must include appropriate financial incentives along with meaningful changes in behavior for both physicians and the hospital. JVs and comanagement arrangements meet these criteria without requiring physician employment.

JVs and comanagement arrangements are proving to be highly successful at aligning incentives between hospitals and physicians. These models, often pursued in combination, are especially useful when improving the efficiency and coordination of care for all components of a particular service line, such as oncology, cardiology, or orthopedics.

# JOINT VENTURES: ALIGNING INCENTIVES THROUGH SHARED OWNERSHIP

Hospital–physician JVs can be developed for everything from practice management services to cardiac catheterization labs, diagnostic imaging, ambulatory surgery, radiation therapy, and most other outpatient services. Recently, this model has been used to form accountable care organizations. JVs are characterized by joint funding by the hospital and physicians, shared control, and common participation in overall management. The basic forms, structural options, and benefits and challenges of JVs are presented below.

Shaped by economic goals and legal limitations, two JV structures have become most prevalent. The *equity JV* includes shared owners of a for-profit entity. The *contractual JV* is virtual, encompassing a relationship defined by contractual terms where interests are aligned but ownership is not shared. While multiple alternatives exist within these two categories and can be refined to meet the specific strategic objectives of the JV, the following examples highlight the main considerations in choosing between an equity JV and a contractual JV.

## Equity JV Models

An equity JV is characterized by the shared investment and risk between the hospital and physicians that solidifies the commitment to the success of the relationship. Ownership models encourage a long-term relationship and strongly align incentives among the partners, who can have equal or different ownership shares. Regardless of ownership distribution, each party can be offered a significant role in the management of the JV.

Under an equity JV, the hospital and physicians create a legal entity that offers specified services or facilities. Each party's ownership percentage is determined by how much it invests in relation to all other investors. The investment can be cash, equipment, the value of an existing business, or other valuable assets. Often, the hospital or physicians will contribute an existing business, such as an ambulatory surgery center (ASC) or imaging center, and the other party will make a cash contribution, essentially buying into the existing service or facility. The ability to buy or sell ownership in the venture is strictly controlled to protect all investors.

However, an equity model may not be appropriate for all JVs. For example, physicians often have difficulty making a meaningful capital contribution. While management can be structured independently of the equity ownership, providing a significant financial return to the physicians without a significant equity investment is challenging. Also, a JV may have difficulty retaining earnings for future growth and investment because earnings are typically taxable for the partner physicians but tax-exempt for the hospital. Without retained earnings, the partners could be exposed to capital calls (additional mandatory investments) to meet future investment needs. Furthermore, when the hospital is contributing an existing business to the venture, physicians frequently balk at the valuation or at paying for a business that, arguably, they helped build through previous referrals.

In addition, hospital executives and board members may not be willing to give up control of a lucrative service to the extent required for success under the JV model. Unless hospital leadership can be persuaded to share control, physicians may not be willing to enter into the JV. Further, if the hospital is located in a state with certificate-of-need (CON) requirements, establishing a new JV entity may be difficult. Obtaining a CON for the venture usually involves long delays and is likely to frustrate the participants. These are all reasons to consider a virtual or contractual JV.

### Physician-Owned Hospitals: Going, Going, Gone

Recent changes in the environment for physician-owned hospitals deserve special mention. Many physician-owned hospitals are jointly owned by a community hospital or not-for-profit health system and community physicians. Interest in this form of JV grew rapidly in the last decade, and many of these whole-hospital JVs are achieving outstanding results in cost containment and care coordination. However, the Patient Protection and Affordable Care Act—the law that was intended to improve outcomes, reduce costs, and enhance the efficiency of healthcare delivery, among other things—bans the development of new physician-owned hospitals and puts tight restrictions on existing hospitals that include physician owners. The law is intended to curb alleged overutilization by physicians who are also owners, a very real problem under production-based reimbursement. The end result is that hospitals are permitted to own physician practices (in most states), while physicians are barred from having an ownership interest in hospitals. Such barriers to economic integration may be removed over time as population-based reimbursement becomes prevalent, but for the near term, new hospital JVs that include physician owners are prohibited.

## Contractual JV Models

While physician ownership requires a commitment from the physicians, it is not always essential to develop a committed working relationship between a hospital and physicians. A contractual relationship can provide a similar sharing of risk and rewards and thus create a strong incentive for the physicians and hospital to work toward mutual goals. A contractual relationship may also be faster to initiate because it involves a lower up-front investment by physicians and fewer legal requirements.

The *time-share lease* is one example of a contractual JV. Under this model, the hospital builds a new outpatient facility, such as an imaging center. The hospital funds the entire cost of developing the imaging center and leases all or part of the center's capacity to a group of physicians. The lease can include space, equipment, staffing, and supplies, all based on the fair market value (FMV) of such services. For example, if the annual lease rate for the facility as a whole is established at $1 million and a medical group needs half the capacity, the group's lease rate would be $500,000. Physicians who have leased a block of time from the imaging center perform procedures and bill patients and payers for the services they provide, including technical services. A time-share arrangement between the hospital and physicians offers a means for the hospital to guarantee a long-term relationship with specialty physicians and for the physicians to share in technical revenue without making a major investment. While the center would not have a hospital–physician board, a joint advisory committee could be established to allow the physicians to have a role in management. And during their block lease time, the physicians are responsible for management of the service.

Contractual JV models provide hospitals with the predetermined revenue stream they need to justify investments in new services. At the same time, the financial rewards to the physicians and their role in management can be structured very much like those in an equity JV.

## Structural Options of JVs

Regardless of the service provided through a JV, the hospital and physicians must agree on the key terms of the relationship. Hospitals should develop a JV policy that defines when the organization will consider a JV, the usual terms under which it will develop a JV, and the degree of flexibility for each of the terms. The following main structural elements of potential JVs should be identified and defined:

- ◆ Corporate structure
- ◆ Ownership structure
- ◆ Leadership and management structures
- ◆ Physician participation

Each of these elements is discussed below.

### Corporate Structure

Key considerations for the corporate structure include the tax implications, limits on the number of shareholders, and complexity of the structure. A *limited liability company (LLC)* is often the best option for hospital–physician equity JVs because of its treatment of liability and tax issues. It is a pass-through entity for federal income tax purposes, although many states impose a small tax. An LLC has no restrictions on the character, number, or classes of owners, and liability is limited for members. An operating agreement spells out operational details.

A corporation can be taxable as a C corporation—meaning double income taxation at both the corporation and the shareholder level—or as an S corporation, where the corporation is a pass-through entity for income tax purposes. The main drawback of S corporations is that they cannot have corporations as shareholders or more than one class of stock.

A *limited partnership* is also a pass-through entity for income tax purposes and has no restrictions on the character, number, or classes of limited partners. The limited partners have limited liability, but the entity must have a general partner whose assets are liable if the partnership defaults. A second limited liability entity, such as an LLC or corporation, is often developed to act as the general partner, thereby adding to cost and complexity.

### Ownership Structure

A hospital should determine the preferred ownership structure for JV opportunities prior to discussions with physicians. Examples of key considerations for the hospital include its willingness to take a minority position and the possibility of offering a management company ownership in the venture. Other factors to consider include the following:

◆ All capital contributions to the JV must be valued at FMV (cash at face amount, other assets according to appraised FMV).
◆ Ownership interests must be proportionate to the amount contributed.
◆ Contribution of cash or property to the venture is generally a nontaxable event, except for the following:
  – Receipt of property (including cash), other than interest in the venture in exchange for the party's contribution, causes a recognition of gain (but not loss) measured by the value of such cash or other property received.
  – An equalizing payment of cash back to a contributing party is taxable to the recipient.

## Leadership and Management Structures

A tax-exempt hospital must maintain voting control over all policies and actions that could affect the organization's tax-exempt purposes. Beyond this basic point, key questions about JV leadership and management include the following:

◆ What are the appropriate leadership and management structures, including their size and composition?
◆ How should the members of leadership and management be determined?
◆ What special leadership and management provisions, if any, should be considered to protect the hospital's tax-exempt status?
◆ What issues should require supermajority or unanimous approval?
◆ Should the power to decide specified issues revert to the owners?
◆ Under what conditions can the JV be dissolved or its business revert to one of the owners?
◆ What rights need to be reserved for certain investors?

An LLC can be managed by all of its members (owners) or by one or more managers who may—but need not—be members. Management details are set forth in an LLC's operating agreement. A physician-controlled medical advisory committee can be useful to manage the clinical operations of a JV. Key management questions include the following:

◆ Will the hospital manage the JV's operations, or will a separate management structure be developed?
◆ Will the physicians be involved in operational or clinical management decisions? To what extent and in what manner?
◆ What is the correct structure to establish a shared service agreement for support services from the hospital?
◆ What services is the hospital willing to provide through a service agreement?

## Physician Participation

JVs can be used to solidify relationships with current medical staff members or to draw in new physicians from competing facilities. They can be structured with individual physician investors, with a newly created physician entity, with an existing medical group or groups, or with a combination of these participants. When planning a JV, the hospital must define both the strategic and financial objectives of the proposed venture. Strategically, long-term partnership and competitive implications may point to a select group of physician investors, while near-term financial needs may require investment from many more physician. If minimum financial needs cannot be met without sacrificing strategic objectives, potential JV participants are all better off deferring plans for the venture until both financial and strategic goals can be realized. Key questions related to physician participation include the following:

- What requirements must be met to be a physician owner?
- Will a noncompete agreement be required?
- Which physicians or groups should be involved?
- Can a fair, market-based, legally compliant arrangement be crafted without alienating key physicians?
- Who are the key physicians, and will they participate?
- How will the medical staff react to the JV?

## Benefits and Challenges of JVs

At the most basic level, JVs offer opportunities for hospitals and physicians to collaborate for mutual benefit. For physicians, this benefit is most often defined as financial return. However, participation in JVs also allows physicians to diversify their revenue base, gain a voice in facility operations, and explore additional collaborative arrangements with the hospital or physicians who are part of the venture. Hospital partners, on the other hand, tend to focus on the strategic implications of the venture, including expanding market share, attracting other physicians, and building trust and respect between the hospital and the physician community.

While the JV can be a potent tool in promoting integration, designing and implementing a deal entails significant risks:

- **Failure to launch:** Negotiating the details of a JV is often contentious. Physicians rarely understand that hospitals operate in a complex legal and regulatory environment that limits how a deal can be structured and how compensation is determined. Capital requirements, profit distribution, sharing of control, design of exit strategies, and operating policies can all reveal major differences between the hospital and interested physicians in terms of perspective and perceived needs. If not managed carefully, these differences can result in the termination of discussions, often after months of effort. The frustration associated with this outcome can seriously damage the hospital's credibility among physicians and can be a step backward, instead of forward, for health system alignment.

- **Failure to thrive:** Perhaps the greatest risk to physician relations is a JV that falls short of projected financial performance. While the hospital can take a long-term perspective and respond to an additional capital call if the venture struggles, the physicians expect the return on investment that was projected in the offering and are rarely interested in contributing more money to cover losses. Failure to meet expected returns is often taken personally by physician investors and can seriously damage their relationship with the hospital. Developing fact-based, conservative pro forma financial statements to minimize the risk of underperformance is clearly important.

- **Failure to adapt:** Even when a JV has been successful, financial results can deteriorate over time, and shifts in the strategic and political landscape can turn a winner into a loser if necessary changes are not made. The most common reasons a JV may fail to adapt are physician owners' blocking needed operational modifications, restrictive transfer arrangements, and a lack of buyback and unwind provisions. For example, a surgical group aligned with a competing hospital may want to buy into another hospital's successful ASC and move their cases, but doing so requires the approval of the existing surgeon investors. They refuse, concerned about losing a competitive advantage. Without a call (mandatory buyback) or similar provision in the investment agreement, altering the participants or services offered within a JV may be impossible.

- **Collateral damage:** Creating a JV can have a significant downside in terms of medical staff relations. Antagonism can potentially arise from anyone who is not offered a share in a JV. Primary care physicians may complain because most JVs involve specialty services and are limited to physicians in those specialties, and they may feel excluded because they don't have the high incomes that allow investment in a JV. If one specialty group forms a JV with the hospital, other groups in the same specialty may feel angry and slighted. If the hospital works with surgeons on an ASC JV, gastroenterologists may complain that they are being ignored, and so on. The hospital obviously needs to manage these varying perspectives and clearly communicate its policies regarding JVs. Statements such as the following can help:
  - The hospital's priorities for JVs are return on investment and strategic value.
  - All proposed projects that meet the hospital's investment criteria will be considered.
  - The hospital will be flexible in structuring JV relationships with interested members of its medical staff.

- **Reduced revenue:** Hospitals entering into a JV with physicians must be cognizant of the overall financial impact on the organization. A JV can result in a reduction of revenue for the hospital, because many of the JV's cases may be pulled from the hospital and the JV's reimbursement will likely be less than what the hospital would have previously received. Thus, not only does the hospital have to share the profits generated from each case, but it must share a lesser amount than it would have received if the case had remained in an out-patient department of the hospital. An impact analysis (i.e., an analysis of the impact of the JV on the hospital) is an important component of the decision process when evaluating a JV opportunity.

JVs between hospitals and physicians have been around for decades and have effectively promoted positive hospital–physician relationships. At the same time, the risks and limitations noted above indicate that JVs should not be considered the sole element of a long-term physician integration strategy.

## COMANAGEMENT ARRANGEMENTS: EMPOWERING PHYSICIANS THROUGH SHARED CONTROL

Under a comanagement model, the hospital and physicians jointly own a company that is contracted to manage day-to-day operations and conduct long-term planning for a specified service line. Cancer, cardiology, neuroscience, and orthopedics are among the most frequently comanaged service lines because of their strategic importance to many hospitals and the opportunities available under physician management. Hospitals generally pursue these arrangements to engage physicians in reducing costs and improving quality. By sharing both management and financial responsibilities, the goals of the hospital and physicians are aligned to enhance the delivery, operational performance, and quality of the service line and to facilitate the development of new service lines. Structural options, common funds flow arrangements, and keys to success for comanagement arrangements are presented below.

### Options for the Structure and Scope of Comanagement Arrangements

#### Ownership and Leadership

A comanagement arrangement creates shared organizational decision making through a joint leadership and ownership structure. While the legal relationships can be structured in a number of ways, a common option is to create a jointly owned management corporation, with physician investors and the hospital each holding a portion of the governing responsibility. Because the investment required to create and operate such a corporation is often limited to consulting and legal expenses, buying in is more affordable for physicians than buying into a JV, which often involves owning hard assets. Ownership of the management company can be split either equally or with majority ownership held by either the hospital or the physicians. Alternatively, the hospital may choose to allow physicians to own 100 percent of the management company, or the hospital may simply contract with an established medical group for management services.

In the example in Exhibit 7.1, ownership of the management company is held by two medical groups, some independent physicians, and the hospital. Creation of the management company requires an initial investment from each owner, with the level of ownership commensurate with the owner's level of investment. In this example, the hospital may own 50 percent of the management company, Medical Group A and Medical Group B may each own 20 percent, and the independent physicians together may own 10 percent. Profits are distributed based on percentage of ownership.

### Scope of Responsibilities

Comanagement arrangements often include one or more medical directors, an operations director, and an outcomes measurement coordinator. Responsibilities of the management company may include the following:

- Development of the service-line strategic plan and operating and capital budgets
- Management oversight of the staffing, equipment, and supply and purchasing plans

**Exhibit 7.1  Sample Management Company Organizational Structure**

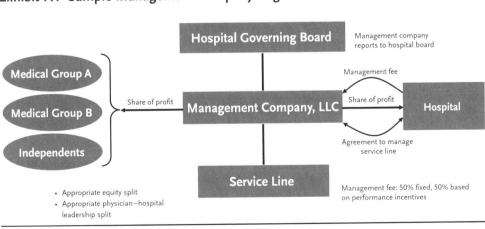

- Negotiation of the service arrangements, including hospital-based services (e.g., anesthesiology, radiology, pathology)
- Approval of payer contracts
- Development of care protocols and quality management
- Case management, including discharge planning
- Creation of improvement policies and marketing strategies

Exhibit 7.2 presents an example of the scope of services that a management company could provide. If the physician partners are relatively sophisticated and have competent management skills, the management company can assume broader administrative responsibilities for the service line. For instance, the management company may employ some service line personnel, such as the service line director, clinical liaison, and others, and may play a larger role in managing ambulatory services that were previously under hospital administration. Conversely, if physician participants are independent of one another and lack management resources, fewer responsibilities will likely be given to the comanagement organization, at least initially. Regardless of the range of responsibilities of the management company when it is first created, the goal is for it to assume responsibility for coordination of the entire service line, including inpatient, outpatient, and physician services. Some situations even warrant having the management company take responsibility for the planning and development of the service line itself.

## Common Funds Flow Arrangements

The management company receives payments for (1) the time and expense required to manage the service line, and (2) the improvements made in financial and operational indicators. Physicians thus have financial incentives to participate in service line management, reduce costs, avoid readmissions, eliminate unnecessary services, and comply with patient care protocols. The basic payment arrangements are discussed below.

### *Payments for Management Services*
The management company receives a fee from the hospital for providing administrative support to the service line; the hospital and participating physicians agree in advance on the services to be included in the comanagement arrangement and set the fee for providing those services. This fee can include costs for physicians and administrative staff, operating costs of the management company, and, in some instances, staffing and operating costs of the service line itself. In many cases, the management company provides physician administrative services only, compensat-

## Exhibit 7.2 Scope of Management Company Services

- **Performance tracking:** Assist the hospital in implementing performance measures designed to improve quality, service, efficiency, and financial performance.
- **Quality assurance:** Perform peer reviews and continuous quality improvement.
- **Training and education:** Train and educate staff assigned to the service line to foster improvements in overall quality, efficiency, and effectiveness.
- **Patient-centered care:** Develop and implement a work plan to improve patient and family communication and education throughout the care process.
- **Throughput and care management:** Implement comprehensive patient care pathways, including standard order sets, daily goals, and post-discharge care continuity plans.
- **Lean processes:** Work with the hospital to streamline the admission process and eliminate documentation duplication.
- **Financial stability:** Investigate causes of adverse performance. Review and make recommendations for improving financial results.

- **Operating room (OR) efficiency and supply standardization:** Implement an OR efficiency program centered on evidence-based process and supply standardization, including evidence-based vendor and product evaluations. Design a tool for in-surgery implant and instrumentation decision making.
- **Contracts, leases, and purchasing:** Evaluate and make recommendations to the hospital about contracts, leases, and purchases, including equipment, instruments, operating supplies, outside services, and repairs.
- **Emerging technologies:** Evaluate and make recommendations to the hospital regarding the quality improvement and investment soundness of emerging technologies.
- **Planning and business development:** Assist in strategic, financial, and operational planning for future services. Assist the hospital in new program planning and development, including exploring the feasibility of a postoperative hospitalist program for the specialty. Support physician recruitment, succession planning, mentoring, and education.

ing the physician partners for the time they spend serving in medical directorship roles and on committees that focus on quality, efficiency, and program development. Typically, the management company pays an hourly rate to physicians serving in these roles, with the rate set at FMV. When the management company employs administrative and other service line personnel, it is reimbursed for salaries and other expenses, which include a small overhead payment. These fees are collectively referred to as the fixed portion of compensation.

### Incentive Payments

The management company's incentive payments are based on achieving specific quality and efficiency measures determined in advance by the hospital and physicians participating in the comanagement arrangement. The best metrics are objective, can be influenced by physician behavior, and drive improvement goals. The metrics usually span the quality, patient experience, and operational and financial goals of the service line. Examples of performance metrics include

- medication reconciliation,
- medical record compliance,
- patient satisfaction (overall),
- patient satisfaction (pain control),
- interval from admission to surgery,
- operating room (OR) turnaround time,
- OR first-case on-time start rate,
- reductions in specific complication rates,
- lowering of readmissions, and
- achievement of outcome measures.

Exhibit 7.3 presents an example of the incentive payments provided through a neurosurgery comanagement arrangement. In this example, incentive compensation is contingent on achieving three or four metrics in each of the following areas: quality, patient satisfaction and education, operational excellence, clinical process standardization, and program development. Each metric has a threshold and target level that determines the physician payment. The full amount of the target payment is awarded for improvements at or above the target level, while improvement between the threshold and target levels results in a 50 percent payout to physician partners.

## Office of Inspector General Guidance on Comanagement Agreements

Advisory Opinion 12-22 of the US Department of Health & Human Services Office of Inspector General (OIG 2012) addresses an existing comanagement arrangement between a rural hospital and a cardiology group. Under the arrangement, the group manages the hospital's four cardiac catheterization labs; recom-

## Exhibit 7.3  Incentive Payment Example

| Item | Reporting Interval | Weight | Threshold * | Target ** |
|---|---|---|---|---|
| **Quality** | | | | |
| Postoperative Infections/Complications | Quarterly | 3% | $ 3,000 | $ 6,000 |
| Risk-Adjusted Craniotomy Mortality Rate | Quarterly | 3% | 3,000 | 6,000 |
| 30-Day Readmission; Related Conditions | Monthly | 4% | 4,000 | 8,000 |
| Quality Subtotal | | 10% | $ 10,000 | $ 20,000 |
| **Patient Satisfaction and Education** | | | | |
| Patient Satisfaction Aggregate Score – Craniotomy | Quarterly | 5% | $ 5,000 | $ 10,000 |
| Patient Satisfaction Aggregate Score – Spine Surgery | Quarterly | 5% | 5,000 | 10,000 |
| Preoperative Spine Education Class for Patient | Monthly | 5% | 5,000 | 10,000 |
| Monthly Patient Care Staff Education | Monthly | 5% | 5,000 | 10,000 |
| Patient Satisfaction and Education Subtotal | | 20% | $ 20,000 | $ 40,000 |
| **Operational Excellence** | | | | |
| Preoperative Patient Documentation Readiness | Monthly | 5% | $ 5,000 | $ 10,000 |
| Block Utilization/Scheduling Efficiency | Monthly | 5% | 5,000 | 10,000 |
| First-Case On-Time Starts | Monthly | 5% | 5,000 | 10,000 |
| Initiate Online Surgical Scheduling | Monthly | 5% | 5,000 | 10,000 |
| Operational Excellence Subtotal | | 20% | $ 20,000 | $ 40,000 |
| **Clinical Process Standardization** | | | | |
| Create, Update, and Track Compliance to Order Sets | Monthly | 10% | $ 10,000 | $ 20,000 |
| Create, Update, and Track Compliance to Care Pathways | Monthly | 10% | 10,000 | 20,000 |
| Standardize Case Preference Cards and Instrument Trays | Monthly | 10% | 10,000 | 20,000 |
| Clinical Process Standardization Subtotal | | 30% | $ 30,000 | $ 60,000 |
| **Program Development** | | | | |
| Develop Spine Center Operational Plan | Onetime | 5% | $ - | $ 10,000 |
| Complete Bundled Payment Analysis and Application | Onetime | 10% | - | 20,000 |
| Develop Resource Utilization Report Cards | Onetime | 5% | - | $ 10,000 |
| Program Development Subtotal | | 20% | $ - | $ 40,000 |
| **Total Incentive** | | 100% | $ 80,000 | $ 200,000 |

\* Threshold performance represents an improvement from baseline and results in a payment of 50 percent of the total possible incentive.

\*\* Target performance represents full performance and results in payment of the full incentive amount.

mends equipment, supplies, and devices; and provides strategic planning, medical direction, staff development, and other services. Advisory Opinion 12-22 is the only OIG opinion that specifically addresses comanagement arrangements. It provides useful guidance about terms of compensation in comanagement arrangements and the inclusion of safeguards against the reduction of services and the inducement of referrals.

Under the arrangement, the hospital compensates the group with a guaranteed fixed fee and a potential performance-based payment. The performance-based payment is capped and based on achievement of employee satisfaction (5 percent), patient satisfaction (5 percent), quality (30 percent), and cost-saving (60 percent) measures. Thus, the comanagement arrangement includes a gain-sharing component through cost savings that accrue to the hospital. Most measures in the performance-based payment use three levels of possible compensation: 0 percent is paid if no improvement is made over the status quo prior to the arrangement, 50 percent is paid for minimal improvement, 75 percent is paid if the middle benchmark is achieved, and 100 percent is paid if the highest benchmark is achieved.

The arrangement prevents the inappropriate reduction or limitation of services in the following ways:

- Cost-saving measures were developed by a team composed of members of the group, other members of the hospital's medical staff, a nurse manager, and members of the hospital administration.
- A third-party utilization review firm monitors the clinical appropriateness of procedures performed in the cardiac catheterization labs and ensures that the arrangement does not adversely affect patient care.
- The hospital and group collaborated to select a single vendor for stents to reduce costs, but the cardiologists adhere to clinical guidelines developed by the American College of Cardiology, and all commercially available stents and balloons are available for use by the cardiologists.
- The performance-based payment is contingent on the cardiologists not stinting on care, increasing referrals, cherry-picking desirable patients, or accelerating patient discharges.
- A significant performance-monitoring infrastructure is in place.

The arrangement prevents the inducement of referrals through the following:

- Compensation paid to the group does not vary according to the number of patients treated.
- The performance-based payment rewards the achievement of specific satisfaction, quality, and cost measures—not additional volume.
- The duration of the agreement is limited to three years. The OIG noted that it would expect quality and cost measures under the arrangement to be subject to change over time, to avoid payment for improvements achieved in prior years.

## Benefits and Challenges of Comanagement Arrangements

Comanagement arrangements are gaining in popularity because they are effective and encourage hospitals and physicians to work together to achieve greater patient satisfaction, improve access, reduce costs, and enhance clinical outcomes. Exhibit 7.4 summarizes some of the benefits of a comanagement arrangement for hospitals and physicians.

On the downside, most of the financial, operational, and political issues associated with any JV apply to comanagement arrangements. Perhaps the greatest challenge is ensuring that physicians enter into a comanagement arrangement with realistic ideas about the time required and the financial return. Specifically, physicians (1) can expect reasonable pay for managing the service line, (2) should not expect compensation for time devoted to the leadership and management of the partnership, and (3) are likely to receive relatively modest incentive payments, even if most goals are met. Early on in the planning process, physicians should be educated about the level of incentive payments they can expect. With proper consideration, comanagement can be viewed as a valuable strategy to transition both physicians and hospitals to the next generation of payment methodologies and care management rather than as an income maintenance strategy for physicians in the near term.

Selecting the right group of physician partners for a comanagement initiative is another key element for success. While allowing any member of the medical staff in a given specialty to be a partner may be expedient, doing so is likely to reduce the success of the initiative. Important criteria for partners in the service line include

- a reputation for quality,
- an interest in improving clinical performance at the partner hospital,
- an ability to work with other physicians and management staff, and
- understanding and sharing the organization's vision for the service line.

The hospital must be willing to focus on alignment efforts with the physicians who are most capable of making a difference and achieving the goals of the management company, even at the risk of antagonizing nonparticipating physicians. The physicians selected to participate as members of the management company should be those who are prepared to put in the required effort, can influence the behavior

**Exhibit 7.4 Hospital and Physician Benefits of a Comanagement Arrangement**

| Partner | Benefits |
| --- | --- |
| Hospital | ◆ Offers a cost-effective and collaborative alternative to employment for the integration of specialists<br>◆ Fosters the development of tools and mechanisms to improve the quality of services<br>◆ Establishes a direct line of input from physicians on service-line growth strategies, technological advances, and performance improvement ideas |
| Physician | ◆ Pays physicians for decisions that significantly affect efficiency, quality, and satisfaction<br>◆ Provides an economic benefit to physicians while allowing them to preserve practice independence<br>◆ Provides a recruitment tool to groups that hold an ownership interest in the management company |

of other clinicians, and seek service-line improvements that mutually benefit the physicians and hospital.

Occasionally, comanagement arrangements are established for service lines that include both employed and nonemployed physicians. In these situations, inclusion of employed physicians in the management company is appropriate if they meet the criteria described above. A portion of the employed physicians' compensation may come from the time they contribute to the management company. However, hospital-employed physicians usually do not own an equity position in the management company.

Legal and regulatory concerns are, of course, a significant part of planning a comanagement initiative. Legal counsel is critical to ensure the comanagement agreement is properly structured to reduce legal or regulatory exposure. Although a thorough description of the legal obstacles of comanagement arrangements is beyond the scope of this chapter, comanagement arrangements are notably affected by the Stark Law, Anti-Kickback Statute, Civil Monetary Penalty Statute, prohibition on inurement and private benefit, and False Claims Act. The requirements can seem daunting to the unacquainted, but a growing number of arrangements comply with all of them, and they should not be seen as a barrier to properly structured arrangements. In general, ensuring the following will limit legal exposure:

◆ All aspects of the transaction priced at FMV
◆ Savings shared only for substitution or standardization of equivalent quality products
◆ No rewards for limiting services or reducing length of stay
◆ No steering of less desirable cases to other providers
◆ No adjusting results to achieve performance targets
◆ No payment that is affected by the volume or value of referrals
◆ Limited contract duration (e.g., three years)

## A LOOK TO THE FUTURE

The future of JVs and comanagement arrangements will be shaped in large part by payment reform initiatives that are currently under way. A complete discussion of the movement toward value-based payments is presented in Chapter 11; the key messages are that population-based payment is likely to become the dominant form of reimbursement, most of the country will take many years to get there, and the rate of change will vary significantly among markets. Healthcare organizations must assess how rapidly value-based payments will penetrate their specific market, because this critical factor will affect strategic planning, particularly the evaluation of JV and comanagement opportunities.

## Joint Ventures

Generally, JVs are created as money-making enterprises that depend on fee-for-service revenue for profitability. However, JVs that are able to adapt their profit-making models to align with value-based payment systems stand to be very successful. For example, several joint-ventured ASCs are doing very well under bundled payments. The best-positioned JVs will learn to leverage the efficiencies and quality of their operations with payers and large employers.

In an effort to contain costs, purchasers of healthcare services are increasingly creating "narrow network" options for their beneficiaries that limit provider choice, especially for elective procedures. By offering unparalleled value or, similarly, by offering bundled episode pricing, joint-ventured ASCs can negotiate with such payers to be exclusive providers of certain procedures within a geographic radius. Well-managed JVs are poised to participate and succeed in these types of payer arrangements. They can gain profitability despite lower service volume per case by increasing commercial patient reach and exclusivity or benefit from shared savings under a bundled arrangement. For hospitals, these kinds of JVs also become important to consider as technological advances continue to push previously profitable services out of the hospital and into the hands of physician competitors on the ambulatory side.

## Comanagement Arrangements

Comanagement arrangements are ideal in a value-based reimbursement world because they typically focus on reducing cost and improving quality. They lend themselves particularly well to combination with bundled payment models, which are gaining ground among both commercial and government payers for episodic care.

Under a bundled arrangement, payments for the professional and technical components of a surgical procedure or acute clinical episode are combined as an incentive for hospital–physician collaboration. The payer typically receives a warranty that any complications of care or readmissions would not merit additional reimbursement for a specified period of time following discharge. Because the bundled price is based on historical utilization, if hospitals and physicians successfully improve the quality and efficiency of their services, limiting care complications, the payment may result in an available savings pool to be shared.

Comanagement arrangements not only provide the vehicle for compensating physicians for their time and energy in jointly managing the process of improving service line value, but they also supply a mechanism for variable compensation based on outcomes. The shared savings or gain-sharing programs that will be part of many bundled payment programs may serve as part or all of the variable compensation provided in a comanagement arrangement.

## THE BOTTOM LINE

The keys to success in JVs and comanagement arrangements are similar, but they are not identical. A notable difference is that JVs need to show an attractive return on a significant financial investment, whereas comanagement projects require a small investment but must compensate physicians for their time and for meeting performance targets. Successful, long-term relationships with physicians in either JVs or comanagement initiatives

- allow for flexibility in structuring an ownership or buy-in model;
- permit collaboration in leading and managing all aspects of the arrangement, to ensure physicians have a voice in the venture or service line;
- seek ways to expand the arrangement over time to further enhance mutual benefits;
- include succession planning as a leadership responsibility, to ensure new physician leaders are developed and included in the arrangement over time; and
- are open to restructuring or winding down an unsuccessful venture in a timely manner, without recriminations.

## REFERENCE

Office of Inspector General (OIG) of the US Department of Health & Human Services. 2012. "OIG Advisory Opinion No. 12-22." Issued December 31. http://oig.hhs.gov/fraud/docs/advisoryopinions/2012/AdvOpn12-22.pdf.

# CHAPTER 8

# Integrated Systems and Accountable Care Organizations: Finding a Fit

*Terri L. Welter*

ALTHOUGH THE DETAILS of healthcare reform are still emerging, it is clear that payments will increasingly be based on value and efficiency and that clinical integration is the key to future success. (See Chapter 11 for a discussion of payment reform initiatives and implications.) *Clinical integration* refers to the coordination of patient care across conditions, providers, settings, and time. It focuses on care that is timely, effective, efficient, equitable, and centered on the patient. The Patient Protection and Affordable Care Act (ACA) identified the characteristics required of provider organizations to be accountable for quality, cost, and overall care for a designated group of Medicare beneficiaries. The ACA officially defined the accountable care organization (ACO) as the model intended to bring hospitals, physicians, and other providers together to better coordinate care and reduce costs. The new requirements for clinical integration will include

◆ an array of providers qualified to contract for and provide all needed healthcare services to a defined population;
◆ sophisticated management systems, including electronic health records (EHRs), financial controls, and operations monitoring and improvement;
◆ the use of clinical protocols and demonstrated best practices in medical management;
◆ a closely coordinated delivery system, including alignment of hospital and physician incentives; and
◆ access to capital required to create the integrated system and manage risk-based arrangements.

A review of these requirements reveals straightaway that past efforts at integration, such as joint ventures, medical directorships, IT support, and even physician employment, fall far short of the collaborative structures that will be needed in the coming years. ACOs are expected to bring providers together to participate in value-based payment models, including the Shared Savings Program (SSP) and population-based payments (PBPs). This chapter focuses on the core elements of ACOs that will drive meaningful alignment with physicians and discusses how to determine the best fit for a given organization in the emerging environment of ACOs.

## THE BASICS

Simply put, an ACO is the legal structure an organization needs to participate in the shared-risk payment models currently being evaluated by Medicare. ACOs are, in fact, intended to accept and manage financial risk for medical services, whether the arrangement is global payment, PBP, or capitation. The Centers for Medicare & Medicaid Services (CMS) will continue to refine standards for ACO designation, and both the Department of Justice and the Federal Trade Commission (FTC) will be providing guidance that will clear the way for the next generation of shared-risk payment arrangements.

The government definition of an ACO is "a group of health care providers who give coordinated care [and] chronic disease management, and thereby improve the quality of care patients get. The organization's payment is tied to achieving health care quality goals and outcomes that result in cost savings" (HealthCare.gov 2013). ACOs are also being formed to manage commercial, Medicaid, and Medicare Advantage populations as the healthcare reform market matures. Clinical integration is the key to moving toward alternative value-based payment mechanisms, and major improvement opportunities are well understood. Areas of opportunity on the inpatient side include congestive heart failure, pneumonia, stroke, and ischemic heart disease. For ambulatory care, the initial focus is likely to be on diabetes, coronary artery disease, hypertension, pulmonary and respiratory issues, and musculoskeletal (back, knee, hip) problems.

At the beginning of 2013, more than 250 designated ACOs existed at varying degrees of integration (Muhlestein 2013). Many more organizations are in the process of forming ACOs, and virtually all acute care hospitals across the country are evaluating if, and how, they should participate in an ACO or similar integrated system. Healthcare providers must develop new collaborative business and organizational models to reflect the interdependence required to coordinate care, to achieve clinical integration, and ultimately to contract under a single signature for risk and commercial business. The legal, financial, and organizational relationships among participants in an ACO must ultimately be designed to provide a framework within which the ACO can legally establish the common infrastructure, financial arrangements, and contracts needed to support clinical integration. The essential characteristics of an ACO are highlighted in Exhibit 8.1.

Establishing and managing an effective ACO requires a degree of integration that few provider or payer organizations have so far achieved. Large multispecialty medical groups and health systems that are fully integrated with physicians and have a health insurance component are currently among the types of organization closest to meeting these standards. The challenge is creating a structure that incorporates the necessary expertise of multiple entities, and few communities have progressed beyond the conceptual stages of collaboration. Each entity brings skills and perspectives that the ACO will require (Exhibit 8.2).

## UNDERSTANDING ACO DEVELOPMENT

Evaluating the feasibility of participating in ACO development requires some detailed considerations. The following paragraphs summarize the most important factors.

### Legal Considerations

As a first step in defining an ACO's governance and management structure, understanding the applicable, current legal requirements is critical. In addition to

**Exhibit 8.1  Essential Characteristics of an ACO**

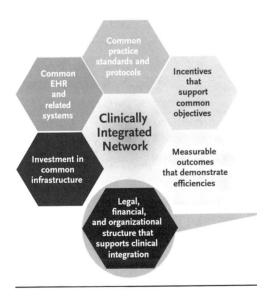

- Network of sufficient size and distribution to support effective management of care across all settings and specialties

- Legal framework and capabilities that allow participants to collectively enter into contracts

- Well-defined governance and decision-making structure

- Alignment of financial incentives among participants toward common objectives

- Single-signature authority for contracts with commercial and government payers

- Ability to accept common financial risk for performance and to internally distribute revenues and allocate expenses

- Sufficient size to support comprehensive performance measurement and reporting

**Exhibit 8.2  ACO Participants and Perspectives**

| Participants | Perspectives |
|---|---|
| Physicians | ◆ Clinical expertise<br>◆ Professional inpatient and outpatient services<br>◆ Other potential assets (ambulatory surgery centers, managed care lives)<br>◆ Ability to affect quality and outcomes<br>◆ Peer review<br>◆ Group management expertise (if partnered with independent practice) |
| Payers | ◆ Provider network<br>◆ Actuarial experience<br>◆ Medical review infrastructure<br>◆ Tertiary and quaternary care contracts in place<br>◆ Experience with drug formularies and durable medical equipment<br>◆ Data systems for monitoring costs and outcomes<br>◆ Data sharing across risk partners |
| Hospital and health systems | ◆ Inpatient, outpatient, and post-acute services<br>◆ Physician network<br>◆ Access to capital<br>◆ System management expertise and experience |

the specific requirements discussed below, each state has laws and regulations that can affect ACO development, including restrictions on the corporate practice of medicine, referrals to other providers, and ownership of ancillary services. The legal concerns that are applicable to all ACO initiatives include the following.

### Medicare

For an ACO that is developed to become a Medicare provider, strict requirements have been established regarding legal structure and governance (Demetriou and Patterson 2011). The ACA dictates that the ACO maintain a formal legal structure that permits it to receive and distribute shared savings payments, to repay shared losses, and to establish, report, and ensure compliance with program requirements. The ACA does not limit the type of legal structure adopted by an ACO as long as the structure is recognized and approved under state law (e.g., corporations, limited liability companies, partnerships, nonprofit organizations).

To guide the development of shared governance, the ACA has two explicit requirements. The first is that at least 75 percent of the governing body be composed of ACO provider/supplier participants or their designees. The second is that the ACO's governing board include at least one Medicare beneficiary. CMS's aim behind the first requirement is to create a structural mechanism that supports the concept that participating ACO providers are aligned because they all have the ability to take part in meaningful decision making regarding the ACO's financial and clinical operations. The second requirement further fosters ACO participant alignment and accountability by ensuring that the Medicare beneficiary population being served has the opportunity to provide input on ACO operations and management.

### FTC Requirements

Whether the ACO is being developed to serve Medicare or commercial populations, the FTC will regulate whether the ACO meets clinical integration standards to ensure that providers are not coming together simply for mutual contracting benefits that might be viewed as anticompetitive. The standards for achieving the clinical integration designation are significant and require substantial coordination and infrastructure within the ACO and among its members. Based on opinions from the FTC to date, a clinical integration model must include at least six key elements:

1. Integration of institutions and practitioners that presents the opportunity for true collaboration and productive sharing of information, reflecting true interdependence
2. Participation of both primary care and specialty physicians, with a requirement of in-network referrals
3. Treatment of a broad spectrum of diseases and disorders, and corresponding clinical protocols
4. Sharing of investment and financial risk, and agreement among physicians to comply with the standards, benchmarks, and protocols put in place by the network
5. Integrated IT, defined as follows:
   - Network participants can efficiently exchange information regarding patient and practice experience.
   - Utilization information can be gathered, analyzed, and communicated to improve treatment quality, rates of utilization, and cost containment.
   - Physician compliance and performance can be documented based on benchmarks and standards of care.
6. Sanctions for noncompliance of physicians and institutions with established structural and operational standards

### Stark Law

The Stark Law essentially prohibits physicians from referring services to any entity in which they have a financial interest. The intent of the legislation was to remove conflicts of interest and the potential for delivery of unnecessary services. However, integration and internal referrals are essential in an ACO environment, and the Stark Law would prohibit any sharing of ancillary revenue with a network of referring providers or a hospital–physician network. To address this concern, CMS and the Office of Inspector General have issued regulations that specify waivers for which ACOs may qualify. The intent is to provide flexibility to ACOs in structuring their operations to share costs and revenues. Because these regulations are evolving, obtaining the most recent regulations directly from CMS is important.

## Organizational Development, Governance, and Management

Beyond the myriad legal and clinical integration requirements for establishing an ACO, the question remains how ACO governance and management will be structured to align physician and hospital partners. An effective way for organizations to begin developing an ACO governance and management structure is to propose a model for discussion that offers a framework for the future state of the ACO. This ACO discussion model should be based on fundamental assumptions, including the following:

- Governance of the ACO will be shared among participating providers.
- Participants will agree to delegate contracting authority and coordination of care by the ACO.
- Participants will contribute capital funding for the ACO's infrastructure and operating expenses.
- Payers will contract directly with the ACO.
- Protocols and clinical practice guidelines will be developed and adhered to.
- The ACO will subcontract with specialty providers when deemed appropriate by its members.
- Participants will commit to develop IT interfaces that enable care coordination.

### Creating Guiding Principles

The degree of integration required in an ACO calls for difficult and complicated decisions about governance, operations, and finances. Providers working to develop an ACO should begin by creating guiding principles that address key questions, such as those shown in Exhibit 8.3.

**Exhibit 8.3 Key Questions in the Development of an ACO**

| Key Topic | Questions to Be Resolved |
|---|---|
| Decision-making guidelines | ◆ Will decision making occur at the local, regional, or system level?<br>◆ What extent of agreement will be required for major strategic decisions? |
| Founding member and participation rights | ◆ Will participating organizations remain independent or merge to form a single entity?<br>◆ Will each member have equal voting rights?<br>◆ Will varying levels of membership be created? If so, what are the rights for each level?<br>◆ How will participant commitment be defined?<br>◆ What participation time frame is required to ensure successful implementation?<br>◆ How will fiduciary responsibility be shared among participants?<br>◆ What are the terms and conditions for withdrawing from the ACO? |
| Market definition | ◆ What market area and populations will the ACO serve?<br>◆ How will the ACO differentiate itself in the market? |
| Operational responsibilities | ◆ Will the ACO leverage existing infrastructure, or will participants jointly agree to develop a new infrastructure to support ACO operations?<br>◆ How will clinical and performance information be shared across the ACO? |
| Provider network and membership development | ◆ According to what criteria will providers be included in the ACO network?<br>◆ How will gaps be identified in the existing ACO provider network?<br>◆ What mechanism will allow independent physicians to be involved?<br>◆ How will providers be removed from the network? |
| Funds flow | ◆ What financial models will be permitted between and among the payers, providers, and enrollees to align incentives?<br>◆ How will surpluses and deficits be distributed? |
| Contracting structure | ◆ How will payer agreements be structured?<br>◆ Which payer partners will be considered?<br>◆ Will the ACO seek compensation for its administrative and medical management functions as well as its clinical services?<br>◆ How will the success or failure of payer agreements be evaluated? |

## Formalizing the Governance Structure

When providers have created a set of guiding principles, the formal ACO governance structure can be designed to reflect and support those principles. There is no best governance and management structure, but the interests of all participating organizations must be represented during the design process. A sample governance and administrative structure is illustrated in Exhibit 8.4.

Regardless of the structure selected, the ACO cannot be a typical hierarchical organization. If the ACO is to be successful, the relationship between participants and committees must be highly matrixed. In fact, each participant's and committee's success is directly linked and completely dependent on the successful functioning of the other participants and committees. Each committee's core functions include collaborative efforts to achieve clinical integration and successful interdependent functioning.

## Redefining Operations

An effective ACO will have a very different set of operating activities from those of today's typical hospital system, medical group, or health insurer. These new activities will be broader in scope, addressing all inpatient and outpatient care, and will apply to a much larger and different population than hospitals or physician groups have served in the past. Addressing this larger scope of activity will be difficult even

**Exhibit 8.4  Sample ACO Governance and Administrative Structure**

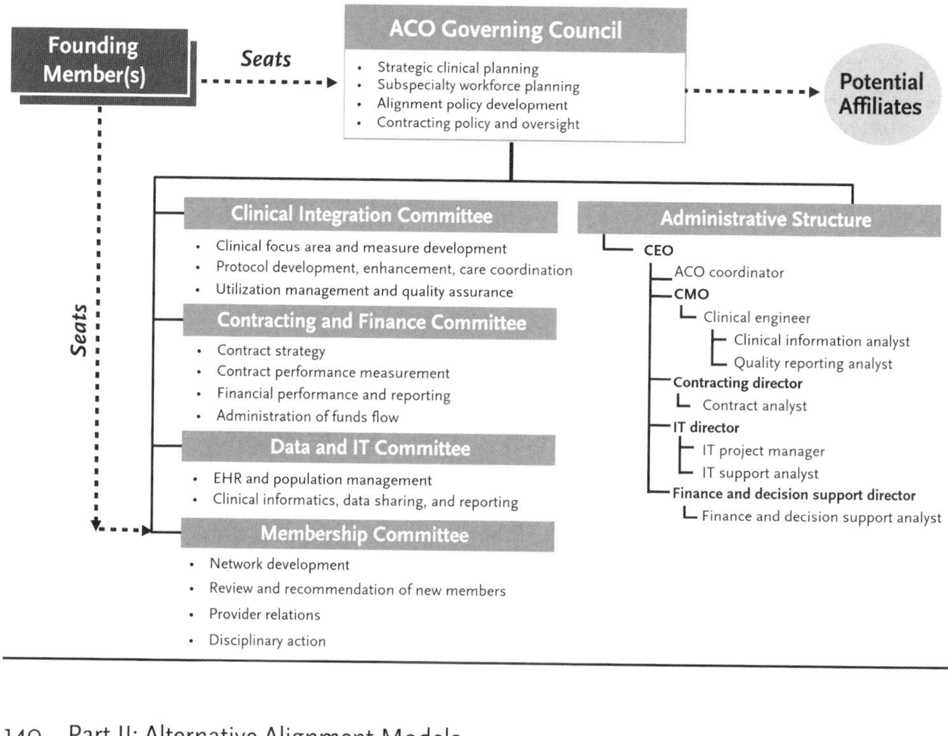

for the most advanced systems. Each organization will bring critical and unique skills to the table. To further complicate the issue, each organization will resist being subsumed under the leadership and culture of another.

For these reasons, serious consideration should be given to the creation of an entirely new entity, one that provides for shared governance and a separate management staff reporting to the ACO board. This structure offers a number of advantages, including

- the ability to create a new culture based on tightly managed delivery of services;
- the opportunity to identify and empower physician leaders to drive the process;
- the selection of initial best-practice partners, because not every provider should be included in the ACO; and
- avoidance of existing bureaucracies, legacy systems, and policies (salary scale, benefits, compliance policies, medical staff regulations) that add complexity and cost without providing significant value.

Because the purpose of an ACO is to change the behavior of caregivers, logically it should be organized independent of existing fee-for-service (FFS)-based organizations and managers. Furthermore, ACOs require a different set of management skills from those normally found in a hospital or medical group. They include knowledge of medical management processes and protocols, provider compensation methodologies, EHR management, population management, actuarial analyses, physician profiling, and targeted client development strategies. A scarce resource will be the integrated system administrator who understands and can oversee clinical integration while dealing with the management structure of the hospital, physicians, and payers. The competition for both physicians and administrators with this skill set will be intense, and compensation will very likely increase substantially in the next few years.

## Payer Contracting

The central purpose of an ACO is to manage healthcare under a value-based reimbursement system. As hospitals and physicians form ACOs and move toward value-based care, they will work with four types of payers pursuing various payment and care delivery models, described in the following paragraphs and summarized in Exhibit 8.5.

**Exhibit 8.5  Payer Types and Prevalent Value-Based Models**

| Payer Type | Prevalent Models |
|---|---|
| Medicare | ◆ CMS shared savings program (SSP)<br>◆ Center for Medicare & Medicaid Innovation (CMMI) Pioneer ACO<br>◆ Patient-centered medical home (PCMH) model<br>◆ Other CMS programs<br>◆ Medicare Advantage |
| Medicaid | ◆ PCMH model<br>◆ ACO initiatives<br>◆ High-risk obstetrics and the NICU |
| Commercial | ◆ Increased pay for performance (P4P)<br>◆ PCMH model<br>◆ Shared risk |
| Employer | ◆ PCMH model<br>◆ High-cost focus areas<br>◆ Wellness programs |

## Medicare

With the introduction of the ACA, Medicare has been laying the groundwork for payment reform in the national market and has served as the catalyst for shifting risk from payers to providers. New Medicare and Medicaid reimbursement rules and initiatives, such as the Value-Based Purchasing Program, hospital readmission penalties, bundled payment demonstrations, and the CMS/Center for Medicare & Medicaid Innovation ACO programs, are incentivizing providers to invest in the care platforms and IT infrastructure necessary to thrive under value-based payment arrangements. Understanding the framework that Medicare has established is helpful, because these initiatives often serve as models for Medicaid and commercial payers and will determine the potential role and responsibilities for provider organizations, including ACOs.

## Medicaid

The very limited budgets in most states have intensified interest in controlling healthcare spending growth and moving state-funded programs away from FFS. The ACA introduced a pediatric accountable care demonstration project beginning January 1, 2012, and lasting five years; much like the Medicare ACO pilot program, the demonstration project authorizes participating states to allow certain qualified Medicaid providers to organize themselves into an ACO for the purpose of receiving incentive payments. Both the federal Medicare program and the state-sponsored Medicaid programs tie provider payments to patient outcomes.

## Commercial

While Medicare and Medicaid program changes are giving providers the most immediate impetus to develop ACOs, many providers see the potential in value-based arrangements with commercial payers to align commercial market incentives with Medicare and Medicaid payment reforms. Such alignment can not only reduce administrative costs but also prevent the conflicting incentives that stem from disparate payment systems. In addition, providers realize that under FFS reimbursement, commercial payers will be the sole beneficiaries of providers' efforts to improve efficiency and coordinate care. More pragmatic reasons to seek ACO contracts with commercial payers include the following:

- Commercial payers can provide some of the resources and support needed to engage in population management.
- Partnership with health plans allows access to payer data that can be used to improve care management systems.
- Commercial payers may be a source of financing for infrastructure and workforce needs that come with care management (e.g., the need to hire nurse navigators).

## Employer

Many ACO initiatives present opportunities to contract directly with large employers and, in particular, to manage health maintenance programs and focus on high-cost patients. Such arrangements could resemble the medical home concept, with specific programs established for high-cost focus areas and wellness. Self-insured employers that use smaller health plans as third-party administrators may also be potential ACO partners. The terms of an arrangement should include, but not be limited to, the following:

- **Membership participation:** Determine what percentage of plan members or employees the ACO will actively monitor and manage.
- **Service offerings:** Outline the health and wellness activities that providers will offer employees.
- **Baseline health metrics:** Identify clinical metrics to be measured among participants.
- **Medical management fee:** Determine a medical management fee, if any, to be paid to providers for service offerings.

As a subset of direct employer contracting, an ACO may contract with its owner hospital(s) and physicians to provide medical care for their employees. Many systems already are self-insured, and many are creating collaborative care pilot programs for their employees.

## DETERMINING THE BEST FIT

While an ACO may appear to offer substantial benefits for providers, hospitals and physician organizations can participate in varying ways, depending on capability, strategy, and culture. Understanding what is needed to be successful is important. Organizations considering ACO participation should follow the steps described below.

### Assess the Organization's ACO Competence

Before defining its role and a detailed strategy for ACO development, the organization needs to take a realistic look at its culture and capabilities as they relate to what is needed to become a successful ACO. Critical factors are summarized in Exhibit 8.6.

### Identify the Most Appropriate Fit

Following its self-assessment, the organization will be able to identify which of the following basic roles is most appropriate for it.

- **Be the aggregator:** Serve as the lead organization in ACO development. Acquire the provider network, provide required capital, negotiate contracts with payers, and manage all clinical and administrative services. Examples include the following:
    - A hospital or health system with a large employed physician network
    - A multispecialty medical group with comanagement responsibility for inpatient services
- **Be a partner:** Participate in the governance and management of a contracting entity. Provide some of the required capital, share financial risk for the contracting entity's performance, and retain operational and financial autonomy. An example would be a hospital and two medical groups that form and

**Exhibit 8.6  Critical Factors in ACO Development**

| Area | Critical Factors |
|------|------------------|
| Operational | ◆ Provider network status (including hospital, primary care, specialty, and ancillary services)<br>◆ Prior planning and development activities with payers<br>◆ Experience with bundled payments<br>◆ EHR implementation progress<br>◆ Experience with clinical collaboration<br>◆ Capabilities of the management team, especially in ambulatory services, IT, and quality metrics |
| Financial | ◆ Availability of resources to support development<br>◆ Contract modeling capabilities to assess appropriate price levels for new payment methods<br>◆ Integrated operational and financial reporting capabilities |
| Political | ◆ Attitudes and risk tolerance of the governing board<br>◆ Relationships with other providers in the region<br>◆ Reputation of the organization in the community, especially with employers |

jointly own an ACO, with each participant retaining its independent corporate status.

◆ **Be a vendor:** Provide clinical services under contract to one or more contracting entities and assume financial risk only for services supplied under contract. Have only an advisory role in governing the prime contracting entity. Examples include the following:
  – A hospital that contracts with one or more ACOs for inpatient services
  – An orthopedic group that contracts with a patient-centered medical home (PCMH) to provide specified services

Not surprisingly, most hospitals, many medical groups, some physician–hospital organizations (PHOs), and a few provider-contracting entities, such as independent practice associations (IPAs), assume they will be the aggregator in their community. This assumption is based on organizational hubris rather than careful planning. The combination of skills and perspective required under value-based payment will limit the number of organizations that can, on their own, be successful aggregators in a given region. The partner role will likely grow in importance as alliances are forged in response to payment reform. The vendor role will remain critical in most areas because many organizations lack the resources or interest to be more active players.

The likely positioning for existing organizations is as follows:

- **Integrated delivery systems:** An enterprise that currently consists of economically integrated hospitals and physicians is obviously best positioned to be an ACO or ACO aggregator. Many integrated delivery systems (IDSs) currently assume some level of risk for a defined patient population and can encompass one or more hospitals, large employed physician groups, home health care or hospice services, rehabilitation services, preventive care, specialty outpatient surgery, and social services. IDSs may also include an insurance plan. A few examples of IDSs in today's healthcare market are Kaiser Permanente, Group Health Cooperative, and Geisinger Health System.

- **Multispecialty group practices:** Multispecialty group practices are generally well positioned to be a partner in an ACO, the key consideration being the identification of a hospital partner. In a market with two or more competing hospitals, positioning the group as a vendor to all may be tempting. This strategy may be fine for some single-specialty groups, but multispecialty groups may not be able to work successfully with hospitals that are competing with each other because of the degree of coordination and collaboration required. However, some practices are developing their own ACOs and subcontracting with other provider partners. This position is appropriate when a group practice has proven experience managing risk, has collaborative hospital relationships, and has the sophisticated infrastructure required to manage an ACO.

- **Physician–hospital organizations:** PHOs are evolving into ACO aggregators in some communities. Historically, PHOs have served as mechanisms by which hospitals and physician groups jointly negotiated contracts with payers. PHOs are typically created through joint ventures between at least one hospital and physician groups (often competitors) that maintain independence but work together to create and deliver more cost-effective patient care services that are marketable to payers. However, to avoid antitrust issues, a PHO arrangement must include primarily risk-based reimbursement methodologies (e.g., capitated reimbursement) for all involved parties (Liethen 2010) or use a cumbersome messenger model. Most PHOs lack the cohesiveness needed to qualify as an ACO, but some already have the sophisticated governance and management infrastructures to support clinical integration, such as Advocate Physician Partners or the Tucson Medical Center, both of which are developing ACOs.

- **Independent practice associations:** Like multispecialty group practices, IPAs are well positioned to be ACO partners. IPAs are associations of independent physician practices that form a corporation to collectively provide services to a managed care plan. Some IPAs have been in existence for decades, and some have even progressed into networks that are undertaking practice redesign, quality improvement initiatives, and implementation of EHRs. As an example, Monarch HealthCare in California is an IPA working to become an ACO through participation in the Brookings–Dartmouth ACO pilot collaborative (Brookings Institution 2011). That said, the majority of IPAs will need to augment their functions and infrastructure to support the level of clinical integration required for ACO partnership and development. Few IPAs have the financial resources, level of provider collaboration, and management capabilities required to take the lead in forming an ACO.

- **Other provider types:** Single acute-care hospitals, high-end tertiary and quaternary hospitals, critical access hospitals, single-specialty group practices, small group practices, solo practitioners, and other provider types (e.g., skilled nursing facilities, home health agencies, kidney centers) are generally best positioned to be vendors to one or more ACOs, but they may also be ACO partners in certain circumstances. An academic medical center may, in fact, be both the lead organization in a local ACO and a partner in or vendor to other ACOs for tertiary and quaternary care.

## THE BOTTOM LINE

In spite of the current fervor surrounding ACOs, provider organizations have a number of viable choices regarding their future positioning. These choices include creating an ACO, participating in a collaborative effort to create an ACO, or becoming affiliated with someone else's ACO. The key points of this chapter are the following:

- Establishing and managing an effective ACO requires a degree of integration that few provider or payer organizations have so far achieved.
- A successful ACO depends on clinical integration to improve outcomes and efficiency, rather than on economic integration to improve profitability.
- The challenge is creating a structure that incorporates the necessary expertise from at least three entities: hospital, physicians, and insurer.
- ACOs require a different set of management skills from those normally found in a hospital or medical group.

Regardless of what they are called, ACOs are a critical element of the transition from volume- to value-based reimbursement systems. Clearly, a value-based reimbursement system will continue to spread from Medicare to Medicaid and private payers. For providers, the ability to assume risk is imperative down the road and a significant opportunity for those who have the systems in place today. Healthcare providers must develop new collaborative business and organizational models to reflect the interdependence required to coordinate care, to achieve federal designation as an ACO, and ultimately to contract under a single signature for risk and commercial business. The question is not if value-based payment will become a significant share of providers' revenue streams, but when.

## REFERENCES

Brookings Institution. 2011. "Accountable Care Organizations Learning Network Toolkit." Engelberg Center for Health Care Reform and The Dartmouth Institute. Published January. https://xteam.brookings.edu/bdacoln/Documents/ACO%20Toolkit%20January%202011.pdf.

Demetriou, A. J., and J. A. Patterson. 2011. "ACO—Legal Structure, Governance and Leadership." ABA Health eSource. Distributed in April. www.americanbar.org/newsletter/publications/aba_health_esource_home/aba_health_law_esource_1104_aco_demetriou.html.

HealthCare.gov. 2013. "Accountable Care Organization." Glossary definition. Accessed April 2. www.healthcare.gov/glossary/a/accountable.html.

Liethen, J. G. 2010. "A Path to Accountable Care Runs Through the FTC." *Law 360* April 28. www.law360.com/articles/163220/a-path-to-accountable-care-runs-through-the-ftc.

Muhlestein, D. 2013. "Continued Growth of Public and Private Accountable Care Organizations." *Health Affairs* February 19. http://healthaffairs.org/blog/2013/02/19/continued-growth-of-public-and-private-accountable-care-organizations/.

# CHAPTER 9

# Information Technology as
# an Alignment Strategy

*Michelle L. Holmes and Asif Shah Mohammed*

As HEALTH SYSTEMS increasingly employ physicians, they also seek to leverage their substantial investments in information technology (IT) as part of an alignment strategy with key community providers, either in addition to or instead of employment. Having a large network of physicians, regardless of employment status, on a similar set of information systems or following a coordinated data strategy can enable a health system to better coordinate care, to mine "big data" to review key cost and quality trends, and ultimately to better position the health system in the community for reimbursement and patient management opportunities. Individual practices and their patients also benefit from access to more comprehensive information and from the economies of scale and scope that allow use of sophisticated technology and functionality the practices might otherwise not be able to implement.

## WHY USE INFORMATION TECHNOLOGY
## AS A STRATEGY?

Over the last few years, the use of IT has come to the forefront as a strategy for physician alignment. In 2006 the federal government relaxed the Stark Law and Anti-Kickback Statute (AKS), enabling health systems to subsidize part of the cost of electronic health records (EHRs) for physician practices. This dispensation led health systems to think of IT as a strategic tool. The American Reinvestment and Recovery Act of 2009 (ARRA) and the meaningful use (MU) imperatives have increased physician practices' demand for sophisticated technology and data exchange capabilities with other provider organizations. Evaluating the viability of

IT as a component of a health system's overall integration strategy must take these environmental developments, as well as the perspectives of both the health system and the physician practices in a particular market, into consideration.

## Health System Perspective—The Road to "Stickiness"

To succeed as an alignment strategy, IT needs to be "sticky" enough that physician practices find pursuing different technology solutions or support models less attractive than continuing to work with the health system's. Proper implementation of EHR technology takes a lot of time and entails significant changes to daily work flows and provider and staff behaviors. Switching from that technology is extremely complicated, so once physicians are using a certain system they will want to stick with it. Therefore, if deployed correctly, IT can serve as an effective tool to achieve meaningful and sustained alignment with physicians.

IT can also be a viable mode of strengthening a relationship in place of tighter integration. For various reasons, exclusive arrangements (leading up to or including employment) may not be an option in a particular market. For example, in a community with only one endocrinology practice but two competing hospitals, neither hospital is in a position to alienate the practice if it chooses to remain independent or to align more closely with the other hospital by renting space in its medical office building. One hospital may, however, provide IT systems, data-sharing tools, or IT services to the practice that enable more cost-effective and streamlined processes, particularly in terms of accepting referrals and delivering acute care. By doing so, the hospital can offer comprehensive services to its patient population and exchange information relating to those services that both improves clinical decision making within the hospital and enhances the overall coordination of care and patient experience.

A health system can also use IT to set the stage for full physician integration, if this is its long-term objective. For example, a health system could initially provide a hosted IT solution, then explore the possibility of migrating providers to a management services organization, which could then lead to a professional services agreement and ultimately culminate in full employment. This progressive approach may be appropriate if practices are hesitant to consider an employment model or if the health system is not yet ready to build and manage a physician enterprise. In either scenario, the health system derives near-term benefit from a relationship based on the provision of IT systems or services while pursuing a more expansive integration model.

## Physician Practice Perspective—Seeing the Big Picture

Often the logic of adopting a hospital-based IT solution is not clear to physicians, and doing so may seem much more expensive than what they can procure from a vendor directly. Most EHR vendors, for example, have offerings that are financially and operationally viable for small, midsize, and large physician practices. A software as a service (SaaS) model requires very little up-front capital investment and typically has affordable per-provider or per-month subscription fees that may be compelling for a small, single-specialty practice. The vendor may even offer content and tools for that particular specialty, resulting in high provider adoption and satisfaction.

However, even after taking full advantage of the technology donation options that are currently available, a health system may still struggle to provide a solution that is competitively priced and appropriately tailored to the visit types and work flows of the practice. An appropriate response to potential skepticism about the IT value a health system can offer focuses on three areas of benefit: data exchange, support, and advanced functionality.

- **Data exchange:** One of the reasons vendors can price systems aggressively for independent practices is that those systems stand alone. That is, with the possible exceptions of national reference laboratories or state immunization registries, information is not being sent to or received from other care providers in the EHR. Although the Continuity of Care Document allows data exchange between systems using media such as CDs or flash drives, such exchange is limited in nature and does little to streamline the ordering and results processes of ancillary services. As described in more detail below, a health system can offer an EHR that is partially or fully integrated with the hospital system and with systems being used by other physician practices, or it can offer exchange tools that enable the practice to retain its system but coordinate more effectively with other caregivers in the community.
- **Support:** A traditional vendor relationship relies primarily on remote assistance once the implementation is complete. Even the support provided during the implementation may be limited; for example, vendor contracts often stipulate fewer than five on-site days for a complete practice management (PM) and EHR deployment. The practice therefore is responsible for most of the day-to-day implementation and training activities leading up to and during go-live. It must also become adept at user support and troubleshooting because vendor assistance is provided only via telephone, Internet, or

e-mail and by individuals who are, more often than not, unfamiliar with the practice and its configuration and work flows. As a component of an IT offering, a health system can provide much more robust customer service, in part because it can hire local or regional resources and distribute the cost of those resources across all of the participating organizations. Instead of five days, it can provide three to four weeks of go-live support, along with structured work flow assessment and redesign assistance as well as tailored and recurring optimization services.

♦ **Advanced functionality:** A physician practice can potentially leverage more sophisticated features and functions from a health system–supported IT program than from a direct relationship with a vendor—either because the less expensive vendor-supplied software does not include the functionality or because the practice does not have the resources needed to configure and implement it. Additionally, many tools offer little or no value if not used in coordination with other healthcare providers in the community. By working with an affiliated health system for IT purposes, a practice is more likely to achieve greater benefit in terms of revenue growth, cost reduction, quality improvement, operational efficiency, and customer service enhancement.

The best way to promote the benefits of a health system IT strategy to a physician practice is to emphasize that the results achieved collaboratively far exceed the results that either organization could achieve independently.


## THREE OPTIONS FOR ALIGNMENT USING INFORMATION TECHNOLOGY

Options for IT as an alignment strategy include (1) providing an ambulatory-focused EHR, (2) establishing a health information exchange (HIE) to support coordination of care among providers who may already have EHRs, and (3) creating an IT services organization that can support the technical requirements of a physician practice.


### Providing an Ambulatory EHR

Hospitals and health systems are becoming increasingly involved in initiatives to deploy integrated EHRs as a means of supporting physician alignment. Deployment may occur through the extension of a core hospital information system as an EHR for physician practices or through enhanced exchange of clinical data between the hospital and community physicians and among physicians. The options for providing ambulatory EHRs include the following, discussed in detail further below:

◆ **Enterprise EHR model:** The hospital implements a single vendor's suite of products to provide access to a patient's medical record in the hospital's inpatient units, outpatient departments, and ambulatory practices (both those it owns and those of affiliated community providers).
◆ **Preferred ambulatory EHR model:** The hospital selects a preferred ambulatory EHR system for physician practices that interfaces with the core hospital system.
◆ **Multiple EHR environment model:** The hospital's system interfaces or connects with multiple EHR systems that practices independently select and operate.

### Enterprise EHR Model

Enterprise EHRs are systems that share a single patient database and common server systems but contain separate application modules for inpatient, ancillary, and ambulatory settings. The shared database integrates the application modules and allows authorized users to access all patient data, which is shared among all providers and facilities.

Organizations using the enterprise EHR model as an alignment option have to make a strategic decision to move toward a single vendor solution. These organizations often regard an EHR solution with a single clinical repository across inpatient and ambulatory settings as providing the greatest potential for improving patient care. The model by which an enterprise suite of products is implemented in physician practices and then extended to other community providers has the following characteristics:

◆ A patient chart that is unified regardless of provider or setting (employed, affiliated, inpatient, ambulatory)
◆ Common patient demographics that can be updated from a single location
◆ Security to maintain privacy of pricing and accounts receivable by practice or unique entity
◆ Integration with ancillary services such as laboratory, radiology, and pathology
◆ Simplified scheduling for inpatient and ambulatory procedures and encounters
◆ Streamlined referral and consultation communications

The use of a single integrated system in the hospital and the physician practice may improve quality and presents an opportunity for the hospital to tie physicians more closely to its services. As mentioned earlier, once a provider is using an EHR, transitioning to a different system is extremely difficult. Additionally, physicians who practice at more than one hospital may value the relative ease of working within an integrated EHR environment and may choose to align more closely with a hospital that deploys a single system.

### Preferred Ambulatory EHR Model

Hospitals that use a preferred ambulatory EHR typically contract with a "best of breed" ambulatory system vendor to provide their preferred system to owned and affiliated community physician practices. The hospital replaces any existing ambulatory EHR products and transitions practices to the preferred solution, which is the only one it supports. To enable data exchange, interfaces are built between the hospital and ambulatory system. In this model, the PM module for billing in the ambulatory setting may not be integrated with the hospital system. Hospitals and ambulatory settings typically decide which data elements will be made available to the physician practices. Key characteristics of this model include the following:

* The hospital's system typically is the ultimate authority for patient demographics and drives the master person index.
* The hospital's system interfaces with an ambulatory system to exchange common data elements, such as demographics, laboratory and radiology orders and results, and hospital reports.
* Multiple instances of the ambulatory EHR can accommodate different levels of data sharing among participating practices, almost all of which limit access to financial information.

One of the key reasons for choosing the preferred ambulatory EHR model is that it allows a hospital to avoid the cost and complexity of transitioning away from its core hospital system vendor to implement an enterprise EHR product. If the hospital already has a core hospital system vendor but the vendor does not have a well-developed ambulatory EHR module, then the preferred ambulatory EHR option would be the least disruptive strategy.

### Multiple EHR Environment Model

The multiple EHR environment model is usually prevalent in organizations that have yet to define their core ambulatory EHR system strategy or whose strategy is still evolving. Under this model, the hospital connects with multiple EHR systems that practices independently select and operate. A hospital typically pursues this model if the community already has an installed base of several ambulatory EHR products. The hospital may decide to work conditionally with the existing products—for example, by interfacing to share data with practices—but it does not provide any additional financial or other support. To execute this model successfully, the hospital will require a robust, flexible interfacing strategy that allows connectivity to multiple ambulatory EHR products in a relatively easy manner. The interfacing strategy could be a point-to-point option or an HIE. The traditional option has been the point-to-point interface, which links each ambulatory EHR to the hospital for the exchange of specific data elements. An evolving strategy is to develop HIEs, which can connect multiple interoperable EHR products, as well as other systems, on a single network. HIEs are discussed in more detail later in this chapter.

The multiple EHR environment model serves as an easy entry point for a hospital trying to partner and exchange data with a large number of small or midsize independent practices that already have an EHR in place. This option is commonly leveraged by smaller community hospitals that cannot afford large integrated solutions. A hospital can achieve the benefits of alignment without having to acquire or employ any physician practices and without having to create the infrastructure to maintain an ambulatory system.

## Selecting an EHR Model

Ultimately, the EHR model a hospital selects will depend on various factors, including

- the existing core hospital system's ability to provide a viable, integrated ambulatory product;
- the prevalence of established ambulatory EHR systems in physician practices;
- the financial resources available to the hospital; and
- the strategic alignment and integration potential within the community.

Exhibit 9.1 presents the advantages and disadvantages of the three different ambulatory EHR models as well as conditions under which each model might be the most appropriate option.

**Exhibit 9.1 Advantages and Disadvantages of Ambulatory EHR Models**

| Key Topic | Enterprise EHR | Preferred Ambulatory EHR | Multiple EHR Environment |
|---|---|---|---|
| Advantages | ◆ Single patient database<br>◆ Easily supports clinical quality initiatives<br>◆ Reduces integration costs<br>◆ Leverages economies of scale | ◆ Focused ambulatory functionality<br>◆ Minimizes options in the market and enables some economies of scale | ◆ Caters to provider preference<br>◆ Supports a variety of price points<br>◆ Implementation and support can be customized to unique practices |
| Disadvantages | ◆ Chart may be cluttered<br>◆ Depends on appropriate use across the health system<br>◆ Requires consensus and standardization | ◆ Requires effective interfacing, which can be costly<br>◆ May result in inadequate provider and patient experiences because of dual-systems approach | ◆ Requires HIE for data sharing and business intelligence<br>◆ Reduces potential for economies of scale (redundant costs)<br>◆ Is costly and resource intensive to maintain |
| Appropriate for | Hospitals that are currently using core systems with robust integrated ambulatory EHR modules | Hospitals that are pursuing a best-of-breed approach and whose physicians will accept a single ambulatory solution | Hospitals that have no preferred ambulatory solution and whose physicians will not accept a single ambulatory solution |

## Moving to Fair Market Value

The relaxation of the Stark Law and the AKS safe harbor, which have enabled donation of EHRs to eligible providers, expire on December 31, 2013. Although various entities are interested in extending donation opportunities at least through the EHR adoption time frame identified in the Health Information Technology for Economic and Clinical Health (HITECH) Act, at the time of this writing it remains unclear whether Congress will grant an extension to the Stark Law exception. When these safe harbors expire, EHRs will need to be priced at fair market value (FMV), which in most cases is substantially more costly than the donation criteria permit. Therefore, organizations providing EHRs under a donation strategy need to contemplate

- whether an established or developing donation strategy will meet the defined regulatory criteria;
- which components of donation pricing may need to be modified to FMV and the impact of this change; and
- what the FMV for similar EHRs will be in 2014 and beyond, given EHR market competitiveness and increasing adoption.

Pricing and sophistication of EHRs used to be correlated—greater sophistication meant higher cost. However, as competition increases and new EHR models enter the market (such as web-based models, SaaS models, and others with prices based on enhancing revenue rather than traditional licensing fees), determining FMV may become challenging. Organizations should consult legal counsel and independent third-party advisory services when developing an appropriate FMV approach.

## Establishing an HIE

All of the ambulatory EHR models described above require a technical solution for sharing data with physician practices, including those with separate ambulatory EHRs. Point-to-point interfaces, which are software-controlled hardware links between each ambulatory EHR and the hospital system, have been the traditional solution in the preferred ambulatory EHR model and the multiple EHR environment model. Some organizations may choose to use an interface engine that is placed between all of the applications to aid in information exchange and monitoring. An interface engine simply leverages a connection that already has the appropriate data and transforms the data for the new application, thereby reducing the time and effort required to design and build data-mapping logic and to test that the data is being delivered as planned.

An evolving alternative to point-to-point interfacing is the HIE. The HIE is a secure, Internet-based network that transmits and receives patient medical record summaries among connected EHRs. A key distinguishing characteristic is that the HIE features a centralized data repository for use by the EHRs connecting to it rather than simply passing data among disparate systems. This characteristic gives an HIE the primary advantage of connecting different EHR products on a single platform. Looking beyond this benefit of flexibility, several hospitals are pursuing HIEs (including those offering the enterprise EHR model) because MU criteria will require the demonstration of interoperability between systems (i.e., EHRs need to exchange data with any certified EHR system) to best support patients who move from one care setting to another. Furthermore, impending changes in reimbursement methods will necessitate greater care coordination.

When a hospital organization decides to evaluate its HIE options, its leadership will be faced with two alternatives: (1) invest in (or start) a private HIE initiative, or (2) wait for a regional or statewide, publicly funded HIE to become available. Because setting up a private HIE requires a large amount of capital, well-funded hospitals and health systems are best positioned to implement this strategy. They are able to create a private HIE that they control through a solution offered by the core hospital system (e.g., Epic, Cerner, McKesson, Allscripts) or a third-party agnostic vendor platform option (e.g., Medicity, RelayHealth, dbMotion). The HIE involves the implementation of a central data repository or community health record for use by the HIE's participants (Exhibit 9.2).

Creating the central data repository involves extracting information from various source systems and transforming and loading it into a consistent database architecture. This process ensures that information defined in each system can be

**Exhibit 9.2 HIE Participants**

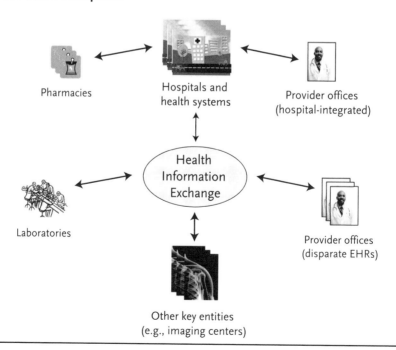

Pharmacies

Hospitals and health systems

Provider offices (hospital-integrated)

Laboratories

Health Information Exchange

Provider offices (disparate EHRs)

Other key entities (e.g., imaging centers)

mapped to similar information in other systems. The HIE may also include services to support population health management and analysis, as well as quality reporting and other types of online analytics that provide actionable data to position the HIE to meet the needs of accountable care. This functionality requires capabilities that are technically feasible only with centralized data architecture, normalized data, and the ability to set up queries easily.

An additional component of the HIE is the collaborative care portal. The HIE portal can serve as a communication tool among physicians and the hospital, allowing clinicians in diverse care settings to see the test results and discharge summaries of all patients and enabling physicians to create new referrals or send quick notes to other members of the care team without disrupting their work flows. As such, the portal can be leveraged to share certain data with practices that are not interested in a higher level of integration. It can also serve as an entry point for an entity that cannot yet connect its system to the HIE but wants to view records populated by other participants.

## Creating an IT Services Organization

If a physician practice is asked what it considers its core competency, it will never answer, "IT support." Many practices are simply not well positioned technologically to support the adoption of clinical IT, business intelligence, and HIE tools. They may not have an IT department at all, let alone one that is of an appropriate size and composition to meet the requirements of an evolving environment that places increasing emphasis on the adoption of sophisticated IT systems. A health system can take advantage of this need and use it as an opportunity to establish a new or stronger relationship with the physician practices in its market. The range of services it can offer is wide and includes the following:

- **Application support:** Provide initial training for new users in PM, EHR, and complementary systems that the hospital sponsors; address ongoing questions and issues; support system optimization and upgrade processes to possibly include customization and template development.
- **Network and desktop support:** Secure, support, and manage a practice's network, desktop computers, and peripherals.
- **Server administration:** Host, secure, manage, upgrade, and administer the application servers the practice uses, enabling a certain level of performance (uptime and response time).

To build an effective structure that provides these and other types of IT services, the organization must carefully define what role each of the various IT staff members will play. Furthermore, experienced end users (or superusers) from various areas, including clinical and nonclinical staff, can be leveraged to enable the practice to provide its own first-tier support, reducing the health system's IT staffing needs and ultimately decreasing the cost allocated to the practices.

Health systems should consider certain key actions for effective support of physician practices, including the following:

♦ Establish standard managerial processes, such as the use of a project management methodology, a vendor management approach with minimum and standard contract terms, and budgeting and tracking tools.
♦ Establish and require minimum hardware and software specifications as well as planned replacement of hardware and routine application upgrades, which are typically lacking in small-to-midsize ambulatory environments.
♦ Use service level agreements for sophisticated IT management processes with community providers to track turnaround times and ensure timely and adequately prioritized support to the physician organizations, so that expectations are accurately set and obligations subsequently met.
♦ Develop an IT department dedicated to the support of the physician practices, to ensure knowledge is shared and provider relationships are managed appropriately.

Well-functioning community IT strategies incorporate a number of roles into either the existing IT department or a specific subunit (separate joint venture structures are rarely used) to ensure that physician needs are appropriately addressed and that the goals and objectives of the health system and the community partners are jointly met. The following staffing positions are key in an IT services organization focused on supporting physician practices:

♦ **Ambulatory IT program manager:** The role of the IT program manager includes the oversight of IT staff and systems, vendor and asset management, MU assessment and remediation, departmental quality assurance and compliance, and execution of the health system's overall IT vision.
♦ **EHR application manager:** The EHR application manager manages the ambulatory EHR system, including its ongoing development and maintenance. He also assists the IT program manager in MU assessment, compliance, and remediation.

- **PM application manager:** The PM application manager is responsible for management, ongoing development, and maintenance of the ambulatory PM system.
- **Business systems analyst:** The business systems analyst provides support related to decision support tools, analytic techniques, data nuances, and methodologies of analysis. She also develops and maintains standard and ad hoc management reports.
- **Interface and systems analyst:** The interface and systems analyst is responsible for the implementation and troubleshooting of clinical interfaces, performance of data mapping and data translations, coordination and maintenance of interface security, and system integrity, compatibility, and standardization.
- **IT help desk analyst:** The IT help desk analyst provides first-tier support to resolve end-user software or hardware issues.
- **Server and network administrator:** The server and network administrator is responsible for the design, installation, configuration, support, maintenance, and evaluation of computer networking and server systems.
- **Database administrator:** The database administrator monitors the performance, reliability, availability, and recoverability of data. He also is responsible for designing and implementing database schematics and conducting regular performance testing and tuning.
- **Application trainer:** The application trainer provides end-user training to ambulatory clinical and nonclinical staff for the required applications.

The number of staff required to support each of these functions varies significantly from one organization to the next. Some resources may be shared with the hospital's IT department, especially in the commoditized areas of desktop support, help desk, and network and connectivity, while specialized resources (EHR application support, training, program management) are typically organized in a separate unit or in a unit with matrixed reporting to IT or physician network development. Because the inpatient and ambulatory modules are integrated in the enterprise EHR model, the number of staff dedicated to the creation and maintenance of interfaces, database administration, and decision support can be lower than in the preferred ambulatory EHR strategy or if physicians were to hire applicable staff independently. Although inpatient and ambulatory training may involve similar principles, organizations typically treat the two environments separately because of the different work flows and system modules involved in each setting. Organizations that use the preferred ambulatory EHR model typically have higher support staffing requirements than those that use the enterprise EHR model, because under the ambulatory EHR model, separate servers and databases need to be maintained for the hospital and the ambulatory systems.

## THE NEED FOR GOVERNANCE—IN ANY SITUATION

Whatever IT option is employed as an alignment strategy, a governance model must be designed. Aspects of governance include board or steering committee composition, leadership and management positions, key bylaws (such as terms and termination), committees and their membership, and responsibilities. The governance structure should include

- a strategic vision that meets the needs of the health system while also supporting the requirements of community providers;
- a governing body with adequate representation from community providers (but typically with no more than 12 members);
- governance that interlocks with other related entities and committees (IT, medical quality, operations) to ensure quality and integration with other key initiatives; and
- A method for prioritizing potential enhancements, changes, or additions requiring capital outlays and addressing them in a fair manner.

As the health system's IT environment matures, the role of the governance body will evolve. Initially, its focus is on questions such as which products will be selected, how they will be supported, and what related services will be offered. Much of the discussion is financial in nature: securing resources, reviewing and approving ongoing requests for add-on products, and addressing variances to budget. The governing body may be supplemented by lower-level committees that focus on more tactical issues about how the system is configured and deployed throughout the enterprise.

Over time, as the health system becomes more sophisticated in its use of the EHR, it gains both a clearer understanding of what the product is capable of supporting and a better sense of what it requires of the product. This experience leads to a more robust dialogue with the vendor about upcoming product enhancements and customizations specific to the health system's needs. As these topics become increasingly important to the IT governance committee, its activities come to include the vetting of product development requests to align with anticipated vendor enhancements and define a specific business case or optimization opportunity.

## THE BOTTOM LINE

Providing IT systems or support is a powerful way a health system can strengthen its relationship with desirable physician practices in the community, either as an independent strategy or as part of a broader goal of alignment and integration. The implementation of these systems or support offerings should not be viewed as the final goal, however; progress is generally slow, failed attempts can mean extensive rework, and the frustration levels may run high among the target audience—physician practice providers and managers. To avoid such frustration, IT system and service goals and their associated metrics should concentrate on improving patient care. This focus is best achieved by setting explicit clinical and operational goals that benefit the health system and practices and by involving physicians in all aspects of planning and execution.

Part III

# SPECIAL CONSIDERATIONS

# CHAPTER 10

# Determining an Arrangement's Fair Market Value

*Kevin J. Duce, Adam J. Klein, and David A. Wofford*

JUST AS THE pace of physician practice acquisitions and employment by hospitals has increased in recent years, so has the level of regulatory scrutiny that these arrangements must face. This scrutiny makes structuring the arrangements in a manner that represents fair market value (FMV) all the more important. As most readers are aware, FMV involves several regulatory requirements, including the Stark Law, Anti-Kickback Statute (AKS), and Internal Revenue Service (IRS) prohibitions against private benefit, and the penalties for noncompliance can be serious not only for the organization but for its leaders personally as well.

This chapter addresses key issues and concepts relating to FMV in two contexts that are frequently encountered in healthcare: physician compensation arrangements (which include not only clinical compensation but also call pay, administrative stipends, and so forth) and physician practice acquisitions.

## BASIC CONSIDERATIONS FOR FMV

Whether contemplating the purchase of a physician practice or crafting a compensation or contractual arrangement, healthcare executives must have a working definition of FMV as well as an understanding of the valuation methods that are used in establishing FMV. FMV is not mere technical jargon; it has real implications for how much the hospital can and should pay, as well as what the hospital is or is not permitted to pay for.

## Valuation Methodologies

Three standard valuation methodologies are used to determine the value of a service, asset, or business. Appraisers must consider all three methods, but occasionally the analysis is limited to two or even just one conceptual approach.

1. **Market approach:** The market approach bases value on an analysis of similar arrangements that have occurred in the relevant market. This approach is the one predominantly used in assessing compensation FMV because reasonably reliable compensation and productivity benchmarks are widely available.[1] It is less useful for practice acquisitions, however, because the terms of practice acquisitions are generally not publicly available and there is no assurance that those arrangements are consistent with FMV.

2. **Income approach:** The income approach considers the present value of future benefits derived from an arrangement (cash flow, typically) and is the preferred approach for practice acquisitions. The challenge is that the acquired practice seldom generates positive cash flows for the hospital. Private practices typically pay out all (or virtually all) available earnings in the form of physician compensation. Given that the buyer often accepts a contractual obligation to compensate physicians at or above historical levels while maintaining and growing the expense structure, the practice is unlikely to generate any excess economic benefit to the buyer. Hence, the practice value ascribed by the income approach is usually zero. Absent the ability to demonstrate value via the market approach or the income approach, either or both parties to a practice acquisition may seek to use the cost approach, described next.

3. **Cost approach:** The cost approach is based on the principle of substitution—that is, it estimates a business's worth based on the costs of reproducing or replacing it. When used to assess compensation FMV, the cost approach and the market approach often yield similar results. In the context of practice acquisitions, using the cost approach as the sole basis for establishing a purchase price can produce a wide range of results, depending on the valuator's methodology. As discussed later in this chapter, this variability is an area of potential risk to the acquiring organization.

## FMV as Applied to Healthcare

The requirement that arrangements be structured in accordance with FMV is by no means unique to healthcare; however, the nature of the hospital–physician relationship presents FMV considerations that do not exist in other industries. The most commonly cited definition of FMV, which was promulgated by the IRS in 1959, is conceptually straightforward:

> The price at which property would change hands between a willing buyer and willing seller when the former is not under any compulsion to buy and the latter is not under any compulsion to sell, both parties having reasonable knowledge of relevant facts. (IRS Revenue Ruling 59-60, 1959-1, C.B. 237, Section 2.02)

This definition is useful in guarding against prohibited excess-benefit transactions, in which a public benefit corporation pays more to a private individual than is reasonable. However, this definition does not specifically address the issue, unique to healthcare, that hospitals have an economic incentive to pay physicians for referrals.

Accordingly, both the Stark Law and the AKS have expanded on the concept of FMV by stating that the price paid must not take into consideration the value or volume of referrals that the physician makes to the hospital; rather, the price must reflect what would occur if neither party were in a position to generate business for the other. In valuators' parlance, one must assume a hypothetical buyer and a hypothetical seller; the hypothetical buyer might be another hospital but in a different market, another physician group, or any other entity that could legally purchase the practice. Similarly, the hypothetical seller might be a group that is similar to the one in question, but perhaps in a different market or otherwise unable to refer patients to the hospital. The Stark Law and AKS further stipulate that, to be FMV, an arrangement must also be commercially reasonable—that is, it must make sound business sense (again, in the absence of referrals) and not be a subterfuge for moving money to physicians without proper justification.[2]

Many readers may find it odd that the notion of FMV is based on an imaginary negotiation between a hypothetical buyer and a hypothetical seller, free from any influence of referrals. After all, most practices have little or no value to a potential purchaser unless the purchaser can realize the benefit of downstream revenue. Therefore, many healthcare executives are not interested in the theoretical underpinnings of FMV and simply want to know how much they can pay without getting into potential legal jeopardy.

Unfortunately, although the regulatory language concerning FMV is strict, it offers very little useful guidance regarding what is an appropriate amount to pay. For example, the IRS definition quoted above focuses on the process through which an arrangement was made but does not comment on what an acceptable outcome of that process is. Additionally, case law offers few insights, because the regulatory agencies and prosecuting attorneys who are charged with enforcing FMV typically will not disclose how they establish FMV or determine which arrangements fall outside it. Because most cases are settled out of court, few ruling opinions exist to guide future decisions. Last, and perhaps most frustrating, valuation and other advisory firms apply different methodologies in determining FMV, with wide variations in outcomes. This variability leaves open the possibility that if an arrangement were investigated, the government's appointed experts could easily arrive at a different valuation from the hospital's. For all of these reasons, it is impossible to know whether a given arrangement would pass muster if it were investigated—a troubling situation that undoubtedly keeps many hospital executives awake at night.

## The Fundamental Tension: FMV Versus Investment Value

The aforementioned challenges in establishing FMV are easier to deal with if the notion of FMV bears some resemblance to the underlying economics of the arrangement; unfortunately, it often does not. Therefore, when evaluating a proposed financial arrangement with a physician, the hospital must approach the arrangement from two different and potentially conflicting perspectives. The first is to determine the investment value, which is the proposed arrangement's worth based solely on the economics of the arrangement. An arrangement's investment value is specific to the parties in question and takes into consideration the synergies that the deal would create—chiefly, physician referrals. This value is often significant and needs to be understood for business planning reasons, even though the hospital cannot pay for the referrals. Second, the hospital must be attuned to the arrangement's FMV, which assumes a hypothetical buyer and seller, excludes consideration for referrals, and has the additional requirement of commercial reasonableness.

The fundamental tension, of course, is that an arrangement's FMV is frequently far less than its investment value to the hospital. Therefore, depending on the relative negotiating leverage of the two parties, the hospital may find itself under pressure to pay more than the arrangement's FMV. This scenario plays out most commonly when a bidding war arises between two hospitals over the same physician group or practice, or when the group or practice faces high costs (whether real or just convincingly asserted) by switching to hospital employment. Distinguishing between the two concepts of value, so that investment value does not influence the perception of FMV, requires an understanding of the issues—not to mention an almost superhuman ability to compartmentalize.

To protect itself from a potential Stark Law violation, a hospital should negotiate the compensation arrangements before it analyzes the economics of acquiring the practice. Doing so will ensure that hospital management did not consider the volume or value of referrals when evaluating and determining physician compensation. While this procedure may seem to defy common business sense, it is necessary because the regulatory environment is so byzantine that the hospital may otherwise unintentionally wander into a consequential regulatory hazard.

## FMV Opinions: A False Sense of Security?

A common misperception among healthcare leaders is that FMV opinions are little more than a cost of doing business. They think that once the deal is done, an adviser with the proper credentials merely needs to "bless" the arrangement with a favorable FMV opinion, and this appraisal will provide the organization with some measure of protection against a potential future encounter with a hostile investigator. Although reasonable reliance on an expert can protect an executive against personal liability, it may not, by itself, provide any protection whatsoever to the organization. The legal protection that an FMV opinion offers to the organization depends entirely on the quality of the opinion—that is, whether it was developed using a sound methodology by a qualified adviser possessing the appropriate experience, knowledge, and judgment. A poorly established opinion may provide some protection to the executive who relied on it but is of virtually no use to the organization. The challenge is that the advisers offering FMV opinions vary tremendously in their qualifications and understanding of the healthcare environment, valuation philosophy, and training, and their opinions vary accordingly. Moreover, valuators have a built-in incentive to please their client by providing the answer that the client is looking for, even if it means bending the rules a bit.

For an executive charged with making a deal happen, this variation in appraisal integrity and practice leads to a perverse incentive. On the one hand, paying less than what a competing bidder is willing to pay may cause an important deal to fall through (and the investment value to be thereby forfeited). This risk is very real, reasonably easy to quantify, and immediate. On the other hand, the organization may pay too much (that is, exceed FMV) and potentially end up in legal jeopardy. This risk is difficult to assess for all of the reasons mentioned above, and in any event it does not have the same perceived level of urgency. Furthermore, because this risk can be mitigated (for the individual, at least) with a favorable FMV opinion, executives have a strong incentive to go "opinion shopping," which creates a very suspicious fact pattern for the hospital if the arrangement is ever investigated.

Therefore, picking FMV advisers on the basis of their leniency is not a wise practice, nor is simply picking one with a good reputation and then relying blindly on his judgment. Executives need to be fairly sophisticated in this area and make informed, well-reasoned decisions, because one never knows how a regulator will judge a given valuation professional's advice. Hospitals need to develop a thoughtful, structured approach to FMV that is well documented and strictly adhered to. Doing so will not eliminate all risk of investigation and a subsequent unfavorable ruling, but it can minimize the consequences of a negative ruling should one occur. A well-planned FMV approach also has the significant side benefit of facilitating consistency across physician arrangements, which in turn makes such arrangements easier to negotiate and manage.

The remainder of this chapter describes FMV considerations for two major categories of financial hospital–physician relationships: (1) physician compensation (which includes stipends for call coverage, administrative services, and so forth) and (2) the purchase of a business enterprise or assets.

## FMV IN PHYSICIAN COMPENSATION ARRANGEMENTS

This section describes some of the key elements to consider when developing a policy regarding FMV in physician compensation, which includes not only clinical compensation but also medical directorships, call stipends, and so on.

### Benchmarking Physician Compensation

Although methodologies for establishing FMV vary, standard industry practice has been to benchmark compensation levels using published surveys such as those provided by the American Medical Group Association; Medical Group Management Association; Sullivan, Cotter and Associates, Inc.; and ECG Management Consultants, Inc., among others. This exercise is part art and part science, and organizations are urged to incorporate the following considerations into their FMV policies.

#### Determine What to Benchmark
Several metrics can be used when benchmarking physician compensation arrangements, including

◆ total compensation,
◆ clinical compensation,

- compensation per work relative value unit (RVU), and
- compensation as a percentage of collections.

These choices are neither exhaustive nor mutually exclusive, and some are more applicable under certain conditions than others. Generally speaking, compensation relative to production (collections or work RVUs) is appropriate for physicians who are able to build a practice and determine their own productivity. Although compensation per work RVU seems to be the most common metric in use, this measure is highly sensitive to geographic and other factors. Industry data also show that compensation actually correlates more closely with collections; the ratio of compensation to collections may therefore be the better metric.

Where compensation-to-productivity ratios are less relevant (as is the case with new physicians who receive an income guarantee or with some specialties that provide a coverage-based service), total compensation or clinical compensation may be useful metrics.

### Choose the Data Source

Next, the organization must determine what data sources it will use for benchmarking purposes. The Centers for Medicare & Medicaid Services (CMS) has affirmed that use of "multiple, objective, independently published salary surveys remains a prudent practice for evaluating fair market value" (CMS 2007, 51015) but does not suggest the specific manner by which survey data should be selected or blended. Organizations should strive for consistency in whatever surveys they use, lest they appear to be selecting a survey or blending methodology based on the results it produces.

### Determine the Rule of Thumb

Although a rule of thumb cannot be used to establish FMV, it can be useful as a risk management tool. For example, many organizations use median total cash compensation from a particular survey or table as an internal safe harbor and conduct additional review only above that level. Determining where to draw the line depends largely on the organization's tolerance for risk, but ideally the decision is informed by qualified experts.

Some advisers take the position that no compensation survey adequately captures all of the relevant dynamics and that the margin for error is therefore high. Consequently, they believe that compensation well above the median (say, seventy-fifth percentile) may satisfy FMV and not require any further explanation. However, the underlying factors causing variation usually can and should be identified when determining FMV. Regardless of the advice given or the specific circumstances, a maximum level of compensation should be established beyond which the organization will not go without significant review and documentation.

In some cases, the FMV limitation may not coincide with the organization's negotiating strategy. For example, the amount that is deemed FMV may be more than the organization needs to pay to get the deal done. When that is the case, the lesser amount should be negotiated.[3] On the other hand, if the physicians are determined to press for a high level of compensation, then the hospital may be genuinely constrained by FMV and may choose to share this fact openly in negotiations. Of course, this information may not persuade the physicians if they have more lucrative opportunities elsewhere.

### Identify Qualitative Factors

In many cases, the organization's internal safe harbor may, for legitimate reasons, be overly restrictive and prevent it from reaching an agreement with a physician who is important to the hospital or community. Examples might include the following:

- The physician's productivity is so high that more than one physician would be required to replace her.
- The requirements of the physician's position are particularly burdensome or necessitate skills that are extremely difficult to find.
- Available benchmark data are not applicable, as might be the case with a highly specialized, luminary physician.
- Recruiting in the specialty has been unusually difficult in the area, and the hospital has documented this difficulty (because recruiting physicians is difficult as a rule).

Although such extenuating circumstances can and do occur, under investigation they may not be sufficiently convincing to result in a favorable ruling. For this reason, such situations should be documented prior to executing the arrangement, to avoid looking as if a rationale was manufactured after the fact.

### Determine When to Seek an Outside Opinion

Every physician compensation arrangement must meet FMV, and a wise practice is to review every arrangement to ensure that it does. However, not every arrangement needs to be examined by a third-party adviser, even though this practice is fairly common. The organization's FMV policy should include guidance on which types of arrangements are sufficiently straightforward that they can be reviewed in-house and which types will require an outside opinion.

To that end, developing a screening methodology to assess the risk of compensation arrangements and assign threshold levels for independent verification is often helpful. Investigators tend to zero in when a total compensation amount is high (perhaps because such information is readily available on an organization's IRS Form 990) irrespective of the underlying productivity or other factors. Therefore, total compensation—whether a dollar amount, a percentile ranking, or both—should be a criterion for determining which arrangements need outside review. Another common criterion is the anticipated or historical compensation relative to productivity. If an arrangement is complex, unusual, or simply outside the organization's expertise, then seeking an outside opinion may be prudent.

## Productivity and Compensation

Although higher-producing physicians generally receive higher levels of compensation, the relationship between compensation and productivity is often misunderstood, and excessive compensation can be the result. For example, one may assume that because a physician is a high producer, her compensation per work RVU or compensation-to-collections ratio should also be above the norm. This viewpoint has a certain logic, because a higher-producing physician makes more efficient use of fixed overhead, leaving more revenue to cover variable operating costs and physician compensation. However, this logic is occasionally taken to an extreme and used to justify, for example, a ninetieth percentile producer earning at the seventy-fifth percentile on a compensation-to-production basis. This approach can potentially result in an unreasonable level of compensation that is not grounded in economic reality or reflected in industry data. The reason is that physicians who receive the highest compensation relative to production tend to be low producers, not high producers. These physicians' compensation is frequently salary based (as is the case, for example, with a new physician on an income guarantee who is still ramping up his production) or consists largely of nonclinical pay (which is reported in the compensation surveys).

## Clinical Compensation Under Cost- and Quality-Based Reimbursement

The widespread emergence of cost- and quality-based payment methodologies adds another layer of complexity to determining FMV compensation. To succeed under these payment methodologies, provider organizations will need to create financial incentives for their physicians that reward cost and quality rather than traditional measures of productivity. Both anecdotal evidence and published research indicate that effective management of readmission rates, chronic diseases, and other episodes of care can result in significant cost savings with no detriment to the quality of care. Rewarding physicians for their role in helping to make such improvements certainly makes sense, but determining an appropriate and legally defensible way to pay their contributions remains a challenge.

Unfortunately, industry survey data are less helpful in this regard than in the traditional fee-for-service environment, for two reasons. First, the data in these surveys are typically up to two years old by the time they are published. Because pay-for-performance compensation arrangements are an emerging phenomenon, they are likely underrepresented in current survey data. Second, benchmarks currently do not provide sufficient information regarding the relationship between compensation- and performance-based incentives that are not tied to productivity, so even if these incentives were well represented in the data, drawing meaningful insights from the data would not be possible.

In the absence of guidance on what to pay physicians under quality-based reimbursement, several practices can be followed to mitigate risk when developing a quality-based incentive plan. In general, until better industry data become available, FMV decisions relating to cost and quality should be guided by the principle of commercial reasonableness. With that in mind, the following guidelines should be considered.

### Alignment of Incentives

If the organization is going to pay physicians for quality or clinical cost improvements, then there should be a clear business rationale for doing so—that is, achieving those improvements should support a tangible economic, strategic, or operational goal. Otherwise, the intent of the payment becomes questionable.

### Equitable Distribution

Similar to the alignment of incentives, any economic benefit for attaining quality or cost targets should be divided among the hospital and the physicians in a manner that reflects their relative investments and contributions. It would make little business sense (i.e., it would not be commercially reasonable) if none of the benefit went to the hospital when it incurred significant costs in developing a physician enterprise and risk-based contractual arrangements.

### Risk and Reward

Performance thresholds should be set at levels that incentivize real improvement, not just reward the status quo. Having small upside-only incentives may be appropriate as a transitional strategy; however, the greater the upside potential, the greater the importance of balancing it with meaningful downside risk.

### Compensation Limits

Upper limits should be placed on the amount of compensation that a physician can earn through cost or quality performance. These limits may evolve over time as the market develops—for example, primary care physician compensation will likely continue to increase relative to specialist compensation—but compensation should not get so far ahead of the market that physicians become outliers.

## Nonclinical Compensation

The same basic principles of FMV and commercial reasonableness apply to nonclinical physician compensation for functions such as call coverage, medical directorships, and other administrative responsibilities. In essence, the hospital is buying the physicians' time, and because the physicians could be spending this time in the practice of medicine, they will want to be paid at a rate commensurate with what they generate in practice. Some physicians will argue that this rate should include the cost of their benefits. Others may contend that if administrative duties are required during normal working hours, then the rate should be sufficient to cover any forgone practice revenues. That rate would be especially high because practice revenues cover overhead and variable costs in addition to physician pay.

Although the opportunity cost of the physicians' time is very real, it does not necessarily constitute a basis for establishing FMV for administrative compensation. In its guidance on methods for determining FMV for physician administrative services, CMS suggests that opportunity cost should not be the sole basis for determining FMV. Furthermore, the FMV of administrative services may differ from the FMV of clinical services (CMS 2007, 51016).

To determine FMV, the hospital should look first to evidence of similar arrangements. These arrangements can often be found in published surveys on call stipends, medical directorships, teaching appointments, and the like. If no such information is available, then calculating an hourly or a per-FTE (full-time equivalent) rate at FMV may be necessary.

To ensure commercial reasonableness, the industry benchmark should reflect the qualifications needed to fulfill the duties of the position, which may be different from the qualifications of the preferred candidate. For example, it may not be appropriate to pay a neurosurgeon her FMV hourly rate to serve on the computerized physician-order-entry committee when a hospitalist could perform that function just as effectively at a lower rate. Similarly, in academic settings, paying a premium for administrative appointments, such as a residency program director, may not be appropriate, even though these positions are usually filled by senior faculty members who earn more from clinical and research work.

## Ongoing Monitoring of Arrangements

Once a compensation arrangement has been put into place, monitoring the arrangement for the lifetime of the contract will be necessary to ensure that it continues to meet FMV. For larger organizations with many physician compensation arrangements, keeping tabs on every agreement is a major administrative task, and failure to do so carries a significant compliance risk that goes beyond FMV. Some common areas of concern include the following:

- Making payments under contracts that have either expired or were never fully executed in the first place
- Not maintaining time sheets for administrative stipends paid on an hourly basis
- Providing fixed-dollar administrative stipends for unspecified responsibilities and performance expectations
- Changing the terms of an arrangement without updating the contract
- Failing to execute cost inflators (e.g., the hospital leases office space to physicians but does not apply annual increases as stipulated in the lease agreement)

Therefore, a major part of an organization's FMV compliance program should include procedures that ensure that compensation arrangements are not only structured appropriately but also administered effectively.

# BUSINESS ENTERPRISE VALUATION

Whereas FMV in physician compensation arrangements is an issue that hospitals must deal with on an ongoing basis, FMV in physician practice acquisitions is much more episodic in nature. It is also more technically complex and nuanced, and for that reason seeking competent professional advice when acquiring a physician practice is recommended. Accordingly, this chapter will not address FMV in practice valuation in great detail; instead, it will highlight several of the key issues that executives should be attuned to. These issues are of particular importance because, in certain markets, purchase prices are being ratcheted up to levels that are unusually high and potentially indefensible.

## The Challenge of Paying for a Physician Practice

When a group of physicians sell their practice to a hospital, the physicians understandably want to negotiate the best price that they can. After having invested their careers in building their practice, they believe they have accumulated tremendous "sweat equity" that the hospital should pay for. Surely, they reason, if the hospital were to build such a practice on its own, it would incur significant start-up and development costs as the practice becomes established. They see the hospital's ability to purchase the practice directly and thereby avoid such costs as clear evidence of the practice's value.

While this argument has a certain logic, it unfortunately does not hold water for FMV purposes. To understand why, it is useful to recall the three commonly used valuation methodologies that were introduced at the beginning of this chapter. As described above, the market approach often is not applicable, given the absence of publicly available information about similar practice acquisitions and the lack of assurance that those arrangements were indeed valued at FMV. The income approach usually results in little or no practice value, because practices seldom generate positive cash flows on their own. Although the downstream revenue makes an arrangement economically viable, the hospital is not allowed to take this fact into consideration.

Because the market and income approaches are rarely helpful in determining what a practice's value is, the usual fallback position is to forgo assigning a value to the business enterprise and instead identify practice assets on which a market value can be placed. This asset valuation is typically accomplished by considering what it would take to replace the assets using the cost approach. As the following section discusses, deciding which assets can be assigned replacement values is not a straightforward process, and the resulting uncertainty poses potential risk for the acquiring organization.

## What Assets Can the Health System Pay For?

Most physician practices have a variety of assets that a hospital may wish to purchase as part of a practice acquisition. These include tangible assets such as real estate, furniture, and equipment as well as intangible assets such as trade names, telephone lists, and the assembled workforce.

Placing a market value on tangible assets is relatively straightforward. An acquiring hospital's or health system's ability to pay for a practice's tangible assets is widely recognized, and valuation methodologies for such assets are well established. Tangible assets have value independent of the practice and of referrals from the practice. Any number of potential buyers might have use for these assets and be willing to pay for them.

The treatment of intangible assets is less clear-cut because experts' opinions in the valuation field differ significantly. Consideration of intangible assets is particularly relevant because the number of arrangements in which hospitals purchase practices for suspiciously large amounts has increased of late, with physician workforce and medical records being the primary drivers of these purchase prices.

The theoretical arguments around the proper valuation of intangible assets are complex but boil down to a fairly simple concept: Whereas tangible assets have value apart from the ongoing operations of a practice, intangible assets do not necessarily have such value. If the utility of intangible assets is tied to a practice that does not have value of its own (excluding referrals, of course), then the value of those assets may be questionable. For example, an observer might reasonably question the value of an assembled workforce in a practice that loses money. Put another way, the fact that an asset has a replacement cost does not necessarily mean paying for that replacement cost is commercially reasonable. If the underlying business is not capable of generating value on its own, then there may be no point in replacing the asset.

The valuation of intangible assets involves unavoidable risk however one interprets the issue. That risk may lead some buyers to forgo a deal that would generate a substantial synergistic benefit. Other buyers may seal the deal but assume a level of risk for their organization that cannot yet be quantified. Because the valuation of intangible assets remains a controversial topic, healthcare executives need to understand, and be comfortable with, their advisers' position on this issue rather than rely blindly on their advice.

## ADDITIONAL CONSIDERATIONS

In addition to the topics just examined, the following questions frequently arise during discussions of physician compensation and business enterprise valuation.

### How Do Purchase Price and Post-Transaction Compensation Relate?

Although the discussion so far has treated physician compensation and practice acquisition separately, they are in fact closely related. As previously stated, when hospitals purchase physician practices, the physicians often receive a richer compensation and benefit package. This has implications for the amount that the hospital can pay for the practice. In the landmark case of *Derby v. Commissioner*, the judge ruled that the financial projections on which a practice valuation is based must reflect the post-transaction compensation. That is, if the purchase price is determined through the income approach using pre-transaction physician compensation, and if the physicians' compensation increases post-transaction, then the hospital will have effectively paid twice for the physicians' pay raise. A regulator would likely consider this a violation of FMV. However, *Derby v. Commissioner* did not provide any guidance about how to address post-transaction compensation increases when the cost approach is the primary determinant of value. Given that the cost approach is used in many (if not most) transactions, a major area of uncertainty remains.

## What If Others Are Paying Large Amounts for Practices?

As mentioned previously, anecdotal evidence suggests that in certain markets, bidding wars are causing provider organizations to pay suspiciously large amounts for physician practices. In such cases, a healthcare executive may have decided to pay a higher price and accept a greater degree of regulatory risk than he otherwise would, to make an important deal happen. Although executives must face such real-world dilemmas, the prevalence of high acquisition prices will not provide them much defense under regulatory scrutiny, particularly if the evidence is only anecdotal and the deals cannot be shown to have been properly assessed for FMV. No one would fight a speeding ticket on the grounds that everyone else on the road was also speeding.

## How Does Community Need Affect FMV?

The discussion so far (particularly in regard to business valuation) has addressed FMV from the perspective of an organization's legitimate business need. However, not-for-profit healthcare provider organizations have a mission that goes beyond mere business considerations and takes into account the needs of the community. Does a hospital's mission to ensure access to needed services have any impact on how FMV is assessed?

Again, opinions in the valuation community differ. One view holds that community need has no impact on FMV; one would not ordinarily pay more based on the fact that the community would suffer if the physician's services were not available.[4] However, the issue could become a factor in commercial reasonableness: A hospital's mission to provide needed services could cause it to enter into an arrangement that it otherwise would have no interest in. Community need could also be used to support a higher payment. For example, paying the replacement cost for intangible assets might be permissible if it means keeping needed services in the community.

Community need is thus another gray area that buyers need to be aware of so that they can make informed decisions and understand the risks involved.

## THE BOTTOM LINE

FMV is a topic of growing interest in the business arrangements between hospitals and physicians, and it will doubtless continue to generate attention in the future. What makes the topic so challenging is that there are seldom clear answers to seemingly simple questions, such as how much a hospital can pay for a physician practice. Despite the absence of any clear guidance and the obvious cost of conservatism in a rapidly consolidating marketplace, the consequences of getting it wrong are severe. While outside opinions can be helpful, healthcare executives need to understand the issues well enough to determine the right balance between achieving compliance and closing important deals.

## NOTES

1. Although the market approach is the most commonly used method in actual practice, the other valuation approaches may be more appropriate, depending on the facts and circumstances.
2. Consider, for example, a hospital that buys a piece of equipment from a group of physicians when the hospital has no legitimate business need for it. Regardless of whether the purchase price was FMV, the deal would not be commercially reasonable.
3. A common view holds that median compensation is always within FMV and that a prudent physician would not accept any amount below this level. If this claim were true, then median compensation would grow dramatically from year to year because last year's median would be this year's minimum. In actual practice, however, median compensation reported in surveys is relatively flat.

4. However, as noted above, if the hospital has documented a history of recruitment difficulties in the specialty in question, a higher price may be appropriate.

## REFERENCE

Centers for Medicaid & Medicare Services (CMS). 2007. "Physicians' Referrals to Health Care Entities with Which They Have Financial Relationships (Phase III)." *Federal Register* 72 (171): 51012–51079.

# Implications of Payment Reform

*Terri L. Welter*

CHANGES IN HOW hospitals and physicians are paid have gained widespread attention, and the issue is generating considerable uncertainty and confusion throughout the healthcare industry. Fee-for-service (FFS) has long been the dominant form of payment for health services in the United States and has played a major role in shaping the delivery of care. Under FFS, hospitals and providers are paid for each of many visits, tests, and procedures. Now that this volume-based payment system is being questioned, other ways of compensating providers are being evaluated and, in some cases, implemented. The concept of value (i.e., demonstrating effective and efficient care at a competitive price) is rapidly becoming a major driver in healthcare. Consumers, employer groups, and government payers are demanding value, and providers are working with payers to move away from volume-based payment methodologies by creating incentives that reward value. Perhaps the most influential factor has been the Patient Protection and Affordable Care Act (ACA), which, among other provisions, includes payment reform designed to transition the reimbursement system to one that is based on value and outcomes. The private sector has also been active, with insurers and providers collaborating to improve quality and reduce costs.

The key messages from recent reform initiatives are the following:

1. The focus on value is here to stay, and payers will continue to develop and refine payment arrangements.
2. Lowering costs and improving outcomes require coordinated care and collaborative management among provider organizations.
3. Providers must become functionally integrated and work closely with payers to be successful.

As value-based reimbursement approaches are developed, providers need to understand these innovative payment structures and how they will affect hospital–physician alignment. This chapter presents a brief overview of the payment methodologies currently being tested, discusses the evolution of payments during the coming decade, and offers guidance on building a competitive payer-contracting capability.

## UNDERSTANDING THE CURRENT MODELS FOR PAYMENT REFORM

The complexity and variation of reimbursement methodologies in the healthcare system can be overwhelming, as multiple payers pay for the same service in different ways. The healthcare industry continues to search for the optimal reimbursement model—one comprehensive enough to address the full range of services while aligning incentives to reward efficiency and quality. Current payment models predominantly use FFS and reimburse based on the volume of service.

Medicare's resource-based relative value system (RBRVS) and diagnosis-related group (DRG) payment methodologies, most often emulated by commercial health plans, are examples of FFS reimbursement models. These payment systems offer little or no incentive to coordinate services to prevent unnecessary care; in fact, they can create a barrier to providing comprehensive, integrated care because they reward individual physicians and hospitals for performing a high volume of separate treatments instead of working collaboratively. Recognizing these shortfalls, virtually all payers—including Medicare, Medicare Advantage, state Medicaid agencies, and commercial health maintenance organization (HMO) and preferred provider organization (PPO) health plans—are piloting innovative payment models. These models take three different approaches: One approach involves specific delivery models; another approach focuses on rewarding specific outcomes; and under yet another approach providers share the financial risk for the cost of care.

Although many models contain elements of all these approaches, recognizing the differences is important to determine which model may be most appropriate in a specific situation. The following paragraphs describe the new payment models in some detail.

# SPECIFIC DELIVERY MODELS

Payment models that use a specific approach to care delivery include the patient-centered medical home (PCMH), the comprehensive primary care (CPC) model, and the Independence at Home demonstration, described in the following sections.

## Patient-Centered Medical Home

A widely discussed model for integrating the delivery of healthcare, the PCMH emphasizes a team-based, patient-centered approach to providing comprehensive, coordinated medical care. Each patient has a primary care physician (PCP) who coordinates the team of professionals needed to ensure appropriate and timely care. A PCMH is used for patients who

- have a chronic disease diagnosis,
- are identified as being at high risk for developing a chronic disease, or
- have an acute condition that requires care coordination to avoid unnecessary complications or duplication of services.

The PCMH model fosters ongoing relationships between the PCP and the care team to ensure that patients receive the education and support they require. Payment approaches vary for the PCMH but have generally evolved to compensate providers through a combination of the following elements:

- FFS for visits and encounters
- One-time or per-patient infrastructure support to cover additional costs
- Pay for performance (P4P) based on quality and either medical spending or utilization metrics
- Shared savings payments if total costs are below the age- and severity-adjusted norms

The PCMH model gained momentum after the ACA included it as one approach to improve healthcare quality and efficiency. States and commercial payers are also collaborating with providers to use PCMH-like arrangements as a foundation for implementing innovative ways to redesign the delivery of healthcare and reduce or control costs. Although state mandates and payer incentives for the PCMH model vary, they all recognize that a mix of initial investments is needed to develop information technology (IT) and human infrastructure.

From the hospital's perspective, the PCMH may appear to generate savings by reducing the volume of facility-based services. While this may be the case, a PCMH approach is well suited to an integrated organization that is preparing for population-based payment (PBP) and can demonstrate successful coordination of care. Under the PBP scenario, a global budget would reward both hospitals and physicians for improving the coordination of care. Other long-term benefits to hospitals include the ability to care for larger populations without the need for additional facility investment, reduced costs as duplicative services or unnecessarily long lengths of stay are eliminated, and avoiding potential penalties or reduced reimbursement for preventable readmissions.

### Creating a Medical Home

Group Health Cooperative in Seattle, Washington, piloted a two-year, whole-practice transformation at one Seattle-area prototype clinic that was centered on the medical home model. The program's 9,200 patient participants experienced 29 percent fewer emergency department visits and 6 percent fewer hospitalizations compared to other Group Health clinics. The results also showed improvements in patient experiences and quality of care and a reduction in clinician burnout. Twenty-one months into the pilot, Group Health estimated its total savings to be $10.30 per patient per month and reported that for every dollar it spent to implement the medical home, it received $1.50 in return.

*Source:* Reid et al. (2010).

## Comprehensive Primary Care

The CPC model is a new approach that builds on the PCMH concept. The Centers for Medicare & Medicaid Services (CMS) CPC initiative is a four-year, multipayer project that fosters collaboration between public and private healthcare payers to ensure comprehensive, high-value, and coordinated primary care. The initiative recognizes the need to support the costs of coordinated care as well as the need to include other payers. CMS provides resources to PCPs for care coordination and works with commercial and state health insurance plans to offer bonus payments to PCPs who are able to better coordinate care for their Medicare patient population.

The CPC initiative tests two models: a service delivery model and a payment model. The service delivery model encompasses risk-stratified care management, access and continuity, planned care for chronic conditions and preventive care, patient and caregiver engagement, and care coordination. The payment model includes a risk-adjusted, monthly care management fee paid to PCPs on behalf of their Medicare FFS beneficiaries. Similar to the PCMH, CPC also incorporates a combination of enhanced FFS and shared savings payments. Initial payments for the first two years of the program will average $20 per beneficiary per month (PBPM), and, as shared savings payments are phased in, the average payment will decrease to about $15 PBPM.

## Independence at Home Demonstration

Another variation of the PCMH approach, CMS's Independence at Home demonstration works with medical practices to test the effectiveness of delivering services at home to improve care for Medicare beneficiaries with multiple chronic conditions. Additionally, the demonstration aims to reward healthcare providers who provide high-quality care while reducing costs. At the time of this writing, 16 independent practices and three consortia were participating in the Independence at Home demonstration, which was announced in April 2012.

## REWARDING OUTCOMES

New payment approaches that reward outcomes include pay for performance (P4P), the Physician Quality Reporting System (PQRS), and bundled payments, as described below.

## Pay for Performance

The label *P4P* is applied to value-based reimbursement models that pay based on quality metrics and outcomes. Under a P4P model, a health insurer or other payer compensates hospitals and physicians according to measurements of their performance compared to process, quality, and outcomes benchmarks. This payment is typically a bonus that the provider receives in addition to FFS compensation. Although most health plans use some combination of quality and cost profiles to determine a provider's or hospital's performance, the approaches used in existing P4P programs vary tremendously. Healthcare organizations and providers must be prepared to explore P4P arrangements as more and more public and private payers pursue this value-based payment strategy.

Current examples of P4P quality measures include common clinical conditions (e.g., diabetes, heart attack, congestive heart failure, pregnancy and newborns), preventive services (e.g., influenza and childhood vaccines), and complications (e.g., surgical infections). As currently structured, P4P rewards individual providers or facilities that meet very specific criteria. As such, P4P does little to promote integration and clinical coordination. However, as measure sets expand to include chronic conditions and broader health status indicators, the need for groups of providers to work collaboratively with the hospital will become more important.

Current P4P programs rely on a limited set of performance measures, and the dimensions of performance vary across P4P programs. Although, as mentioned above, measure sets focus on preventive services, common clinical conditions, and complications, some P4P programs also include measures of patient perceptions derived from satisfaction surveys, and other programs provide financial rewards for investments in health IT. Exhibit 11.1 lists examples of conditions with quality metrics that various reporting agencies are tracking. Two examples of P4P programs, one commercial and one governmental, are described here:

**Exhibit 11.1 Selected Conditions Tracked by Reporting Agencies**

| Condition | The Joint Commission | Hospital Quality Alliance | CMS Public Reporting | CMS/Premier Demonstration | The Leapfrog Group |
|---|---|---|---|---|---|
| Heart attack | X | X | X | X | X |
| Heart failure | X | X | X | X | X |
| Pneumonia | X | X | X | X | X |
| Surgical infection | X | | X | X | X |
| Pregnancy and newborns | X | | | | X |
| Hip and knee | X | | | X | X |

*Source:* Data from National Committee for Quality Assurance (www.ncqa.org).

- **Commercial:** Nationwide, Blue Cross and Blue Shield plans are replacing many future increases to provider reimbursement rates with P4P arrangements. Health systems that are moving to these arrangements must consider the importance of an effective transition period to avoid financial disruptions. A successful transition model contains the following major components:
  - Protection against inflation by including an annual adjustment tied to the medical consumer price index or other agreed-on measure
  - Outlier compensation to pay for catastrophic cases
  - A phased-in approach to P4P metrics that allows time to develop the specific quality improvement initiatives or measurements required by the program
  - Support for implementing systems or IT interfaces to automate the reporting of performance metrics
- **CMS programs:** Many programs being implemented or expanded by CMS will have P4P as a component, and payments to providers and hospitals will depend more on quality and efficiency. One example is the Hospital Value-Based Purchasing Program, which applies to payments for discharges occurring on or after October 1, 2012. Under this program, CMS will adjust DRG rates based on either how well a hospital performs on certain quality measures or how much the hospital's performance improves compared to a baseline period. The higher a hospital's performance or improvement is during the performance period for a fiscal year, the higher its value-based incentive payment for the fiscal year will be.

## Physician Quality Reporting System

The PQRS is a voluntary reporting program for physicians. Under the program, CMS makes incentive payments to physicians who satisfactorily report data on quality measures for covered physician fee schedule (PFS) services furnished to Medicare Part B beneficiaries. CMS publishes the data on a website (www.cms .gov/PQRS) that both serves as an authoritative source for publicly available information and provides CMS-supported educational and implementation support materials about the PQRS. Many physicians are currently participating in the PQRS, and hospital partners need to understand this program and its importance for introducing physicians to measurement and accountability for quality parameters.

## Bundled Payments

Bundled payments reimburse providers with a lump sum for services related to an episode of care or a chronic condition. The lump sum includes payment for both hospital and physician services, and the hospital and physicians are responsible for determining how the lump sum is to be divided. Bundled payments are most often used for joint replacements and other high-cost surgeries.

Bundled payments can be designed prospectively, in which case provider groups receive full payment in advance, or retrospectively, so that claims are paid on an FFS basis and costs for the bundled payment service are reconciled against a total cost target. Under a bundled-payment arrangement, providers can achieve success by reducing input costs and increasing the value of services. Additionally, through gain sharing, providers may receive bonus payments for meeting certain quality benchmarks. Although the scope of bundled payments is relatively small, a bundled-payment arrangement can be an appropriate option for hospitals with one or more strong service lines.

♦ **Bundled Payments for Care Improvement initiative:** In 2011, CMS announced the Bundled Payments for Care Improvement (BPCI) initiative, which allows hospitals to apply to receive bundled payments for certain procedures. Bundled payments can be made under several models of care:
   – *Model 1: Inpatient stay (hospital services only).* The hospital is paid a discounted IPPS (Inpatient Prospective Payment System) payment, and the physicians are still paid FFS.
   – *Model 2: Inpatient stay plus post-discharge services.* This model includes inpatient hospital and physician services, related post–acute care services, and associated admissions.
   – *Model 3: Post-discharge services only.* This model includes post–acute care services and related readmissions.
   – *Model 4: Readmission inpatient stay only.* This model includes inpatient hospital and physician services but excludes post–acute services.
   The BPCI program is intended to give hospitals and providers new incentives to coordinate care, improve the quality of care, and save money for Medicare by lowering the cost of care. Some observers believe that this pilot program is likely to become more widely prevalent under Medicare, including as a feature of accountable care organizations (ACOs). Furthermore, commercial payers are widely testing other versions of this payment methodology. Hospitals that are well aligned with their physicians and are implementing systems that can satisfy the requirements of these programs stand the best chance of successfully adapting to the BPCI payment paradigm.

- **Acute Care Episode demonstration:** The CMS bundled-payment initiatives, and similar projects contemplated by commercial payers, grew out of a successful project called the Acute Care Episode (ACE) demonstration. In the ACE demonstration, five sites took part in a three-year project that tested the use of bundled payments for certain cardiovascular and orthopedic procedures. CMS paid the participating hospitals a lump sum for all Part A and Part B services, including physician services, pertaining to the inpatient stays of Medicare FFS beneficiaries. The hospital was responsible for compensating the physicians and other providers for their services. Cost reductions in the ACE demonstration were achieved primarily by standardizing devices and reducing surgical supply costs.
- **PROMETHEUS Payment model:** The PROMETHEUS Payment model covers the full episode of care and all providers. It distinguishes probability risk from technical risk, and payments are derived using a complex formula based on an evidence-informed case rate (ECR). Health system cost savings are achieved through reduced payments for potentially avoidable complications (PACs), adjusting for the severity and acuity of the patient.

Although the cost-saving potential of bundled payments is gaining considerable attention from private payers and the government, reimbursement is often problematic. First, a limited number of appropriate bundles exist, which leaves most of the vast universe of medical services unaddressed. Second, payer savings are achieved primarily by paying less for the average bundle than for unbundled FFS. Providers must therefore reduce the intensity of service, costs, or both to realize any financial benefit. Finally, physician commitment has proven to be weak when the upside to participation appears limited.

### Private Sector Bundled-Payment Arrangements

SSM Health Care–St. Louis and Anthem Blue Cross Blue Shield decided not to wait for Medicare to implement a bundled-payment system. Starting with a single bundled-payment arrangement for total knee replacement, the health system and insurer collaborated to reduce costs while practicing evidence-based medicine and documenting outcomes. The program has expanded to include total hip replacement. This initiative has positioned SSM well in the era of value-based reform, and the organization is poised to increase the number and types of services included in bundles with Medicare.

*Source:* ECG Management Consultants, Inc.

## SHARING RISK

Broadly defined, two approaches are currently used to share risk with providers: shared savings programs (SSPs) and PBP. The key components of each are discussed below.

### Shared Savings Programs

In SSPs, providers, including both hospitals and physicians, are paid on an FFS basis, but if the total costs of providing care for a defined population or for a specified service are lower than expected, the providers receive a share of the savings. In some instances, a portion of the FFS payment is withheld and paid out only if quality and cost targets are met. As with bundled payments, the reward to physicians for achieving savings may not be adequate to drive major changes in behavior beyond the short term. This model also depends on the availability of cost and quality data for the at-risk services as well as agreement on the benchmarks for performance. As a result, this approach is best suited for specialized services and patient populations and is unlikely to be broadly adopted as a payment model.

### Population-Based Payment

Under PBP approaches, providers are paid a fixed monthly amount for supplying a specified range of services to a covered population, subject to maintaining quality and access standards. The providers themselves determine how to distribute the available revenue. PBP systems reward the coordination of care and reduction of costs, but they require a high degree of clinical integration. The challenge of PBP for hospitals, physicians, and other providers is to develop organizations that allow effective collaboration.

Although a broad array of models allow risk sharing among payers, providers, and facilities, the ACA officially defined the ACO as the model intended to bring hospitals, physicians, and other providers together to better coordinate care and reduce costs (see Chapter 8 for a full discussion of the structure and function of ACOs). Many state Medicaid agencies are rolling out various ACO models, and some health systems are using the ACO model to align and integrate the delivery of care among their hospitals, physicians, and health plans.

The move toward PBP is reminiscent of the surge in HMOs and capitation payments to providers that occurred in the late 1980s and 1990s. The previous movement toward risk contracting fizzled largely because of a perceived lack of consumer choice as well as resistance in both the insurance and the provider communities.

Important lessons were learned, however, and given today's economic pressures and changes in the political climate, the transfer of risk away from the government and payers toward providers and consumers is likely to gather momentum. PBP will likely replace FFS as the major payment methodology for providers, but completing the transition will take many years.

Exhibit 11.2 compares the advantages and limitations of shared-risk models with those of the other types of payment models described in this chapter.

---

### A Medical Group Assumes Risk

An 85-physician medical group in the Midwest entered into a risk arrangement with a Medicare Advantage health plan to manage the care of approximately 5,000 members. The group ultimately achieved a medical loss ratio of less than 70 percent and experienced improved care outcomes and patient satisfaction. The group's investments in its population management infrastructure were critical to its success. The group's major efforts included

- Deciding how ancillary or outside revenue will be allocated among group members (e.g., equal shares, based on use, based on ownership),

- implementing a common EHR platform,

- developing data repositories to facilitate the identification of high-risk patients,

- creating a care management department and utilizing trained care management staff to improve the management of high-risk patients, and

- adopting evidence-based medical guidelines to create a uniform standard of care for all providers in their treatment of patients.

The focus on high-risk patients presented the greatest opportunity for reducing costs.

*Source:* ECG Management Consultants, Inc.

---

## Barriers to Shared-Risk Models

Significant barriers to shared-risk models include the following:

- Current legal and regulatory standards make formation of a qualified network a long, complex, expensive, and risky undertaking.

### Exhibit 11.2 Payment Models: Advantages and Limitations

| Payment Model | Advantages | Limitations |
|---|---|---|
| PCMH and related models | ◆ Focused management of high-risk populations<br>◆ High patient satisfaction<br>◆ Facilitates integration across the care continuum | ◆ Requires major infrastructure investments<br>◆ Requires cross-practice coordination and cultural transformation<br>◆ Complicates physician compensation in the multispecialty group setting<br>◆ Medical cost results are still under study |
| P4P | ◆ Simplicity and clarity<br>◆ Focused approach produces results on select measures<br>◆ Current models tie increased dollars to performance measures | ◆ Historically, limited dollars have been tied to outcomes<br>◆ Focused approach limits comprehensive overhaul |
| Bundled payments | ◆ Comprehensive, outcomes-based approach<br>◆ Pilots (commercial and Medicare) focus on high-cost surgical services in closely aligned hospital and physician specialties (e.g., cardiac surgery, orthopedics) | ◆ Complexity<br>◆ Usually pays FFS with a manual shared savings reconciliation process<br>◆ Need to improve outcomes- and cost-reporting capabilities<br>◆ Focused approach limits widespread application |
| Shared risk | ◆ Aligns incentives<br>◆ Major upside opportunity<br>◆ Facilitates integration across the care continuum | ◆ Complexity<br>◆ Requires economic integration to be truly successful<br>◆ Infrastructure requirements<br>◆ Care management sophistication and focus<br>◆ Significant financial risk |

- The challenges of creating effective clinical collaboration, including care delivery and performance metrics, are substantial. To be effective, provider organizations will require a degree of integration that few healthcare delivery systems have so far achieved.
- Many organizations have cultures that are firmly entrenched in FFS, even if their stated strategy includes moving toward shared-risk and population-based payments. As previously noted, the functional differences between FFS and at-risk payment models are significant. Right or wrong, culture trumps strategy, and unless organizational culture is changed, attempts to promote coordinated care will be stymied.

## PREPARING FOR PAYMENT REFORM

It is a challenge to understand even the basics of the many different approaches to payment reform, let alone to figure out what approach to take in a real-world hospital or medical group environment. The core message of all this action is that healthcare is somewhere in the early to middle stages of a transition from FFS to PBP. The path a hospital takes and its speed of conversion will depend on the dynamics of its community and payer market, but hospital–physician integration is clearly a critical enabling element in the transition process.

For the near term, shared savings approaches will remain common because they can reduce costs without changing the FFS base. Over time, however, PCMH projects and other PBP initiatives, including Medicare Advantage, will see continuing successes. During the coming years, hospital-led integration will increase, creating many more organizations that are capable of accepting and managing PBPs. Medicare and Medicaid will lead the way in transferring risk to provider organizations, while private payers will learn from the government programs and follow with their own PBP initiatives. SSP payments will be subsumed under more widely based PBP for well-organized provider networks.

Clinical integration—the coordination of patient care across conditions, providers, settings, and time—is key to moving toward value-based payment mechanisms. The new requirements for clinical integration with physicians are likely to include

- a high degree of interdependence between and among providers and hospitals,
- a full panel of PCPs and specialty physicians with required in-network referrals,
- integrated IT (EHR) and robust reporting capabilities,

- basic competence in population health information,
- clinical protocols across a broad spectrum of diagnoses and procedures,
- sophisticated revenue distribution and compensation methodologies to align incentives, and
- noncompliance penalties for both physicians and institutions.

Taking on financial risk through PBP systems is especially challenging because it gives physicians, hospitals, and health plans responsibilities that are frequently different from their well-established processes. Exhibit 11.3 summarizes some of the interdependencies in risk contracting.

Given these requirements, competencies clearly will have to include physician leadership, practice management expertise, IT capabilities, and financial strength

**Exhibit 11.3 Key Responsibilities in PBP Arrangements**

| Party | Key Responsibilities |
|---|---|
| Physician | ◆ Clinical integration across care continuums<br>◆ Outcomes-driven approach<br>◆ Strong care management<br>   – Referrals<br>   – Inpatient days or admissions<br>   – ED visits<br>   – High-tech radiology events<br>   – Prescription rates of generic pharmaceuticals<br>◆ Strong data collection and analytical capabilities |
| Hospital | ◆ Strong case management<br>◆ Strong data collection and analytical capabilities<br>◆ Hospital–physician integration<br>◆ Efficient and effective ED care management<br>◆ Reducing unnecessary readmissions<br>◆ Implant or high-cost drug expense management<br>◆ High-tech radiology management |
| Health plan | ◆ Linking payment to utilization and quality<br>◆ Bundling individual services within a payment system (e.g., dialysis)<br>◆ Stop-loss and catastrophic case coverage<br>◆ Premium pricing<br>◆ Administrative expense management<br>◆ Strong data collection and analytical capabilities<br>◆ Data sharing across risk partners |

and sophistication as well as a committed network of providers and services. Each of these points is addressed in other chapters of this book, but preparing for payment reform will also require the following steps.

## Understand the Payer Market

Some organizations likely have a good understanding of the hospital market and even the physician market in their immediate area. It is less likely that they understand the payer market in terms of how insurance companies measure up with respect to their provider networks, new products under development, data management capabilities, and strategic priorities. Hospitals need to meet with, and learn from, the insurance companies' senior managers.

Current market dynamics—the type and rate of change that can be foreseen in reimbursement and how organizations should respond—should also be considered. For example, many small hospitals now receive charge-based reimbursement. Commercial payers in most markets are likely to move—if they haven't already—toward inpatient case rates, which will require many changes in how the small hospitals operate. Along similar lines, many hospitals are moving to provider-based reimbursement for employed physician networks. Payers, including Medicare, can and will modify compensation levels as they deem appropriate. The current payment differentials will likely not be maintained for long, because they will be either revised downward or replaced by PBP.

## Assess the Organization's Role

Before an organization develops a detailed strategy for coping with payment reform, it needs to take a realistic look at its culture and capabilities as they relate to value-based payment. The organization should consider the same critical operational, financial, and political factors as those for participation in an ACO (see Exhibit 8.6 in Chapter 8).

If an organization is not yet ready to shift aggressively to value-based reimbursement, then of course it should do everything possible to maintain volume-based contracts while introducing quality and efficiency metrics and promoting coordination of clinical services. These efforts will help the organization to develop needed skills and begin to educate stakeholders. However, organizations should take care not to drive down volumes while stubbornly sticking to an FFS reimbursement policy. Otherwise, the hospital and physicians do the work while the payers get the rewards.

## Develop an Explicit Strategy

After an organization considers its role, selecting objectives and specific initiatives is much easier. Too often, however, hospitals focus on creating the structure and governance of a contracting entity, such as an ACO, while paying scant attention to the functional requirements of coordinated care. Instead, an organization should prepare a payment reform strategy that addresses three categories:

- ◆ Clinical coordination
- ◆ Provider collaboration
- ◆ Cost control

If a hospital starts with an initiative that targets these three categories, the organizational structure will emerge as part of the process. Additionally, an organization should not focus solely on measuring quality and documenting outcomes. Providers also need to understand their current costs and pricing structure as well as how they compare to other providers across the portfolio of services. In both the short and longer term, rationalizing payment structures can result in significant gains.

## THE BOTTOM LINE

Payment reform is happening, and the transition to value-based payments is not likely to stall out or disappear. The economic and political pressures on the healthcare system are simply too strong to maintain the status quo. Specifically, shared savings and PBP systems will become significant sources of provider revenue in the coming years. The critical lessons in managing this transition are the following:

- ◆ **Ensure that clinical coordination is the top priority.** A fundamental principle for planning and operations should be to facilitate medical group integration and service line development.
- ◆ **Engage payers in all aspects of planning.** Payment reform requires very different relationships between providers and payers. Today's often contentious relationships must be converted into effective business partnerships.
- ◆ **Inform and involve stakeholders.** Payment reform is a complex process that will entail changes for virtually all participants. Educating all stakeholders, including physicians, board members, managers, and staff, is critical if the needed changes are to be made without major disruptions.

# REFERENCE

Reid, R. J., K. Coleman, E. A. Johnson, P. A. Fishman, C. Hsu, M. P. Soman, C. E. Trescott, M. Erikson, and E. B. Larson. 2010. "The Group Health Medical Home at Year Two: Cost Savings, Higher Patient Satisfaction, and Less Burnout for Providers." *Health Affairs* 29 (5): 835–43.

# Index

Bolded page numbers indicate information found in exhibits and boxes.

Integrated delivery systems for ACOs, 146
Integrated health systems. *See also* Accountable
    care organizations (ACOs)
    average loss per physician, **68**
    as context in discussions, 15
    flexibility needed in, 31, 37
    scope of activities of, 8
    strategy for, 5–6, **7**
Internal Revenue Service (IRS), 167, 169

Joint operating committees (JOCs), 41
Joint ventures (JVs). *See also* Clinical coman-
    agement arrangements
    aligning incentives through shared owner-
      ship, 115–122
    ambulatory surgery centers (ASCs) in, 131
    benefits and challenges of, 120–122
    bundled payments benefiting, 131
    certificate-of-need (CON) requirements,
      116
    contractual JVs, 115, 116–117
    corporate structure, 118
    effective integration strategies, 114
    equity JVs, 115–116
    financial and strategic objectives in,
      119–120
    future of, 130–131
    hospitals' perspective on, 114
    leadership and management structures,
      119
    limited liability companies (LLCs), 118,
      119
    limited partnerships, 118
    overview, 113, 115
    ownership structure, 118
    Patient Protection and Affordable Care Act
      (ACA) impact on, 116
    in physician–hospital organizations (PHOs),
      146
    physician-owned hospitals, 116
    physician participation, 119–120
    physician perspective, 113–114
    physician relationships in, 132
    structural options of, 117–120
    time-share lease, 117

Leadership. *See* Physician organization and
    leadership
Letter of intent (LOI), 22–23

Loyalties, 6

Management structure implementation,
    42–44, **43**. *See also* Clinical comanagement
    arrangements
Managing the transaction
    acquisition feasibility criteria, 21, **21**
    asset purchase, 31
    communication plan, 29–30, **30**, 70
    confidentiality agreement, 22
    definitive agreements, 25–26
    design and documentation for, 21–27
    documents and completion time frames,
      **26**
    financial analyses to include, 20
    getting organized for, 27–28
    implementation plan topics, 27
    letter of intent, 22–23
    multiple group or multispecialty transac-
      tions, 30–31
    project management support, 28–29
    retention, 32
    securing approvals, 32
    term sheet, 23–25, 32
    testing feasibility, 19–21
    transition planning, 26–27
Market approach to valuation, 168, 179
Market position in term sheet negotiations,
    25
Meaningful use (MU) imperatives, 149, 158,
    160. *See also* EHR Incentive Program
Medicaid, **142**, 142–143. *See also* Centers for
    Medicare & Medicaid Services (CMS)
Medical groups, differences between hospitals
    and, 70–71, 78, 84, 86
Medical staff reaction, 16
Medicare, 78, 136–137, 142, **142**, 186, 191,
    193. *See also* Centers for Medicare &
    Medicaid Services (CMS); Fee-for-service
Memorandum of understanding, 22–23
Metrics, physician vs. hospital, 10
Migration path to consolidation, traditional,
    **37**, 37–38
Multispecialty group practices in ACOs, 146

New practices, 69–70
Nondisclosure agreement, 22
No-shop provisions in letters of intent (LOIs),
    23

# About the Editors

**David A. Wofford**

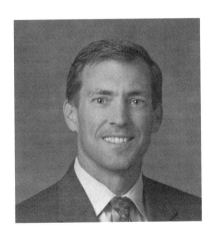

Mr. Wofford is a senior manager at ECG Management Consultants, Inc. Since 1996, Mr. Wofford's consulting career has focused on physician business affairs and hospital–physician relationships. He works closely with medical groups on matters such as group practice formation, physician compensation plan redesign, revenue cycle management, and clinic operations. He advises hospitals on physician practice acquisitions, strategic planning, and the negotiation and development of professional services arrangements with physicians. The breadth of Mr. Wofford's experience provides him with an understanding of the issues related to hospital–physician relationships and affiliations as well as of the perspective and value that each party brings. This understanding, in turn, allows him to develop sustainable arrangements between the two parties. Prior to joining ECG, Mr. Wofford served eight years as an officer in the US Army. He holds a bachelor of arts degree in economics from Duke University and a master of business administration degree from the University of Chicago.

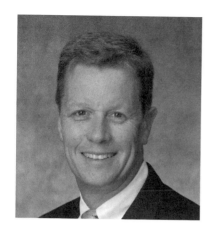

Mr. Messinger is the managing partner of ECG Management Consultants, Inc., and a member of the ECG board of directors. As head of ECG's eastern healthcare practice, Mr. Messinger has extensive experience in strategic and business planning, business development, mergers and acquisitions, and managed care. He assists health systems, academic medical centers, and medical groups with developing and implementing strategies that drive competitive advantage, and he is an effective adviser to boards and executives who are managing the challenges and implications of transformational change. Mr. Messinger has been a featured speaker on healthcare strategy and hospital–physician relationship issues for a variety of professional associations, trade groups, health systems, and physician groups. He has been published in several healthcare journals, including *Modern Healthcare*, *Modern Physician*, *hfm* (a publication of the Healthcare Financial Management Association), *Group Practice Journal*, and *Health Care Strategic Management*. He earned a master of health services administration degree from the George Washington University and a bachelor of science degree in clinical sciences from Cornell University.

# About the Contributors

## Scott F. Burns

Mr. Burns is a senior manager at ECG Management Consultants, Inc. He joined ECG in 2008 with more than 25 years of healthcare experience in mergers and acquisitions and business, strategic, and facility planning. Over the years, his work has resulted in tactics to enhance growth and performance, reduce costs, and improve patient populations' access to needed healthcare services. Prior to joining ECG, Mr. Burns was a director in the health industries advisory practice of a Big Four consulting firm and a director for Tenet Healthcare Corporation's predecessor company, where he was responsible for overseeing acquisition and development activities as well as leading planning and financial analyses in support of transactions and capital investments. Mr. Burns has a bachelor of arts degree from Purdue University in West Lafayette, Indiana, with a concentration in public administration and an emphasis on health services administration.

## Benjamin C. Colton

Mr. Colton is a senior manager at ECG Management Consultants, Inc. He leads ECG's revenue cycle practice. He assists health systems across the country in evaluating, optimizing, and improving their revenue cycle to support enhanced financial performance and operational alignment. He is also an expert on the operational and regulatory requirements for transitioning from freestanding to provider-based billing designation. Prior to joining ECG, Mr. Colton worked with a large multi-provider clinic, where he helped manage billing operations. Mr. Colton holds a master of business administration degree from F. W. Olin Graduate School of

Business at Babson College and a bachelor of arts degree from the University of Washington.

## Kevin J. Duce

Mr. Duce is a senior manager at ECG Management Consultants, Inc. His health-care consulting experience emphasizes hospital–physician alignment and strategy, physician network development, compensation planning, and operational assessments of medical groups and hospital-based services. Prior to joining ECG, he worked at Children's Hospitals and Clinics of Minnesota in the performance improvement department and as a clinic administrator. Mr. Duce has master's degrees in health administration and business administration from the Carlson School of Management at the University of Minnesota and a bachelor of science degree in biology from St. Olaf College.

## John N. Fink

Mr. Fink is a senior manager at ECG Management Consultants, Inc. He assists healthcare provider organizations with strategic and business planning, hospital–physician alignment, new business ventures, and mergers and acquisitions. Mr. Fink is certified as a project management professional by the Project Management Institute, Inc., and received both a master of business administration degree and a bachelor of science degree in finance from Indiana University.

## Jennifer K. Gingrass

Ms. Gingrass is a principal at ECG Management Consultants, Inc. She focuses on physician practice issues, ambulatory operations, process redesign, and hospital–medical group integration. Her practice concentrates on the organizational, strategic, operational, and financial alignment between large, multi-specialty group practices and affiliated health systems to achieve care delivery integration. She is a frequent speaker at American Medical Group Association and Healthcare Financial Management Association industry meetings. Prior to joining ECG in 2004, Ms. Gingrass worked in health and welfare benefits consulting at a global consulting firm. Previously, she provided day-to-day physician practice management. Ms. Gingrass holds a master of science degree in health systems management from

Rush University and a bachelor of science degree, with an emphasis on science–business, from the University of Notre Dame.

## Joshua D. Halverson

Mr. Halverson is a principal at ECG Management Consultants, Inc. He has more than 15 years of experience in healthcare strategic and business planning, hospital operations, and physician organization development. Mr. Halverson previously worked in the healthcare strategy practice of a nationally recognized management consulting firm and as a senior director in an integrated healthcare system in Southern California. He holds master's degrees in healthcare administration and public health from the Carlson School of Management at the University of Minnesota, with concentrations in financial management and quantitative methods.

## Sean T. Hartzell

Mr. Hartzell is a senior manager at ECG Management Consultants, Inc. He focuses on strategic and financial planning, service line development, and hospital–physician alignment with a particular interest in hospital–physician employment transactions. Mr. Hartzell has extensive experience in hospital strategic planning, orthopedic service-line development, physician compensation plan design and implementation, and physician compensation fair market value analysis. Previously, Mr. Hartzell held business development and finance positions at Inova Health System. He received a master of business administration degree from the Darden Graduate School of Business at the University of Virginia and a bachelor of science degree in operations research and industrial engineering from Cornell University.

## Michelle L. Holmes

Ms. Holmes is a principal at ECG Management Consultants, Inc. Her practice leverages her extensive experience in assisting with the implementation of an electronic health record (EHR) in a large, ambulatory healthcare system. With a concentration in curriculum design and implementation of the EHR, as well as the development of population management and decision support tools to enable heart disease and diabetes care, cancer screening, and childhood immunization tracking, Ms. Holmes helps physician groups leverage their EHRs to address strategic and operational challenges. She has master's degrees in business administration and health services administration from the University of Washington, a bachelor of arts degree in health services administration from Eastern Washington University, and a bachelor of science degree in business management from the University of Utah.

## Adam J. Klein

Mr. Klein is a senior manager at ECG Management Consultants, Inc., and the head of ECG's valuation services practice. Since 1997, he has conducted economic damages assessments for taxable and tax-exempt entities as well as valuations and appraisals of business enterprises, physician and executive compensation arrangements, accountable care funds flow arrangements, and capital and intangible assets. Mr. Klein is a certified valuation analyst with the National Association of Certified Valuators and Analysts, a member of the American Society of Appraisers, and qualified by the Institute of Business Appraisers to perform business appraisal reviews. He received a master of business administration degree from the UCLA Anderson School of Management and a bachelor of arts degree in econometrics from the University of Massachusetts Amherst.

## Darin E. Libby

Mr. Libby is a principal at ECG Management Consultants, Inc. His healthcare background and leadership skills give him the experience to solve complex client problems, with specific expertise in corporate strategic planning, hospital–physician arrangements, and medical group financial management. Prior to joining ECG, Mr. Libby worked at Overlake Hospital Medical Center in Bellevue, Washington, where he led an effort to build a new hospital and managed the physician practice division. He also served as the cancer service line administrator at The Methodist Hospital System in Houston, Texas, where he managed the development of a comprehensive breast center and a urology institute. Mr. Libby received a master of health administration degree from Washington University School of Medicine in St. Louis and a bachelor of arts degree from Austin College.

## James W. Lord

Mr. Lord is a principal at ECG Management Consultants, Inc. He is a member of ECG's board of directors and heads the firm's midwestern healthcare practice. He specializes in physician strategy, organizational development, and incentive design. Prior to joining ECG in 1997, he worked in medical group management for a large, integrated delivery system in the Midwest. Mr. Lord's background in operations and strategy provides him with a broad range of skills necessary to evaluate and address difficult healthcare issues. He holds master of business administration and master of health administration degrees from Saint Louis University.

## Curtis A. Mayse

Mr. Mayse is a senior manager at ECG Management Consultants, Inc. He has 25 years of executive-level experience specializing in physician strategy, operational practice assessments, hospital–physician acquisition and integration, and revenue cycle improvement. He is a frequent speaker on practice management and strategy topics and a professor in master of health administration programs. During his previous ten-year tenure with LarsonAllen LLP, he was the national principal in charge of physicians and medical groups. Mr. Mayse is a fellow of the American College of Medical Practice Executives of the Medical Group Management Association and an AAPC certified professional coder. He received a master of business administration degree from Maryville University and a bachelor of science degree in accounting from the University of Missouri.

## Francine D. Merenghi

Ms. Merenghi is a principal at ECG Management Consultants, Inc. She has more than 25 years of senior-level experience in medical group administration in independent and integrated delivery systems as well as faculty practice plans, including experience managing large medical groups and developing and implementing physician-related strategies. Before joining ECG, she provided leadership and strategic and operational direction as vice president of operations for a 350-physician enterprise affiliated with Mercy, a leading integrated delivery system. Ms. Merenghi holds a master of business administration degree from Lindenwood University in Missouri and a bachelor of science degree in business and marketing from Saint Mary-of-the-Woods College in Indiana.

## Asif Shah Mohammed

Mr. Shah Mohammed is a manager at ECG Management Consultants, Inc. He joined ECG in 2008 with extensive experience in information technology (IT) and strategic planning and implementations for large health systems and multi-specialty physician practices. At ECG, his practice focuses on leveraging the use of information systems to address strategic and operational issues related to technology acquisitions and deployments. Previously, Mr. Shah Mohammed worked as an IT operations manager at Gateway Health System, a project analyst at Jefferson Regional Medical Center, and an account manager and consultant for Pacs Pro, Inc. He has a master of business administration degree from Owen Graduate School of Management at Vanderbilt University and a bachelor of science degree in electrical engineering from the University of Rochester.

## Terri L. Welter

Ms. Welter is a principal at ECG Management Consultants, Inc., and the head of ECG's contracting and reimbursement practice. Since 1996, she has worked in the areas of managed care and provider payment, including strategy development, reimbursement, contract negotiations, and operations. Ms. Welter is a frequent national speaker on the topics of evolving provider payment vehicles and accountable care organization development. She holds a master of science degree, concentrating in healthcare administration, from Villanova University and a bachelor of arts degree in preprofessional studies from the University of Notre Dame.